BETTER DAILY
SELF-CARE HABITS

BETTER DAILY SELF-CARE HABITS

Simple Changes with Lifelong Impact

CICELY HORSHAM-BRATHWAITE, PhD

ROCKRIDGE
PRESS

Interior and Cover Designer: Erik Jacobsen
Art Producer: Meg Baggott
Production Manager: Martin Worthington
Production Editor: Ashley Polikoff

Paperback ISBN: 978-1-64876-979-5 | eBook ISBN: 978-1-64876-980-1
R0

To my beloved Charles, thank you for giving my heart a home. Mwah!

CONTENTS

INTRODUCTION

You may have been attracted to this book because you have wanted to develop, practice, and commit to self-care in your daily life for some time but have not quite gotten the hang of it. That makes sense. Knowing what is healthy or helpful is different from understanding *how* to get there. Consider your past attempts at self-care as laying the groundwork for this new paradigm of commitment.

Twenty-five years ago, when I was a stressed-out doctoral student, I happened upon a course called "Extreme Self-Care." I had no idea what that meant or if I wanted to be "extreme" about it, but it seemed like the course could help me get a grip on my life. The course changed my perspective entirely. I learned that I could take active measures to support my well-being and make self-care a lifestyle. Moreover, I realized that failure to practice self-care made the stressors in my life more challenging to negotiate. Since then, I have been on a mission not only to deepen my own self-care practices but also to provide information and inspiration on this topic to my family, friends, and clients. I am proud that those in my sphere of influence count the self-care lessons I have shared as one of the aspects of our relationship they most appreciate.

For a long time, self-care was regarded as something distinct from what mental health professionals offered clients. The topic was certainly not in my graduate school curriculum, nor anything that I read about in my professional journals in years past. The tide, however, has turned: the 2021 Stress in America Survey commissioned by the American Psychological Association recommends "15 to 30 minutes of self-care" per day as an evidenced-based practice to counteract the impact of stress. My profession now acknowledges what change-makers and activists like poet Audre Lorde have long touted: self-care is essential.

It's true that developing new self-care habits will come with its own set of challenges. The good news is that the strategies in this book can be learned by anyone and incorporated into everyday life to make real change happen relatively quickly. This book will assist you in building healthy habits and breaking any bad habits that may be challenging you.

The book is structured to help you move from having the intention to upgrade your self-care to actively creating ongoing habits that can be applied to your daily life. Each habit presented is designed to optimize your success by offering a reliable way to begin, tangible actions that you can implement, and guidance on how to recognize the benefit you derive. You can practice the habits as written or customize them to your liking.

To get the most out of this book, pick a core set of self-care behaviors to incorporate into your life. You will then use the habit trackers to monitor your success. Before you know it, you will have ramped up your self-care across multiple facets of your life.

UNDERSTANDING HABITS

Self-care is all the rage right now. Far too often, however, the popular emphasis on self-care omits the practicalities that bridge the desire to incorporate self-care into your life and the actual practice of self-care on a regular basis.

Taking the desire to practice self-care and making it a reality in your life requires behavior change, and behavior change relies on the power of habit. Consequently, it's essential that you understand the ins and outs of the habit-building process so you can establish and maintain effective self-care habits.

The chapters in part 1 will enhance your awareness of habits by explaining what they are and how they can impact your life. You'll learn how to ensure that the new self-care habits you build are effective, and you'll also get an overview of the facets of self-care that are discussed in detail in part 2.

Take a moment to congratulate yourself for being willing to start this journey and prioritize your self-care. Now, let's jump in!

What Are Habits, and Why Do They Matter?

After you read chapter 1, you will have a clearer sense of what habits are and how they are formed at the behavioral and biological level. You will understand how to spot your own habit patterns. You'll also possess greater knowledge about how bad habits form and why it may have been hard to change them in the past. Once you are equipped with this information, you'll be able to take stock of the habits in your life, and you'll be able to better decide on the habits you'd like to establish and habits you'd like to change. Then you can begin to craft a plan for doing so.

Habits 101

Habits are actions taken repeatedly in the course of your daily life. They start with a cue from the world around you, which you respond to by making a decision to pair a set of actions together into a behavioral chain. The brain's strategy of linking environmental cues together with actions by associating them to one another is called "chunking." An easy way to think of this is as a chain reaction that sets off other actions. For example, taking a deep breath before diving into a pool is an unconscious habit. Seeing the water is the cue, and the act of taking air into your lungs before jumping into the water continues the behavioral chain.

It is tempting to believe that people who regularly engage in healthy habits such as daily exercise or meditation simply decide to create a routine and stick to it. Although this is possible under certain circumstances, it's more likely that they consciously engaged in habit formation—and this is key. Each person has the ability to make meaningful changes in their life when they consciously harness the power of habits.

Here are four guiding principles I have found to be crucial when helping my clients develop self-care habits:

1. Develop a goal.
2. Break down the actions to reach your goal into steps. Start small and add in steps over time.
3. Repeat the habit in the same context and in response to the same cue over and over.
4. Expect bumps in the road and plan for them.

You'll learn more about how to incorporate these principles in chapter 2. Self-care habits developed and strengthened over time will help you create the life you desire. Habits are building blocks for creating a happier and healthier life, because they provide a road map for achieving your goals.

The Habit Loop

In order to make positive changes in your life and create long-term, healthy habits, it's important to understand the habit loop. The habit loop describes a process in which something that happens in the world around you (a stimulus) leads you to engage in a particular behavior (a response). The reward that you get from engaging in that behavior develops a habit. A habit can be negative or positive, can be formed consciously or unconsciously, and can be simple or complex.

My clients enjoy using the acronym **TAG (Trigger, Action, Gain)** to signify this process. TAG is a mnemonic that adds some levity to the process of change by calling to mind a game of tag as a means for achieving a goal. Both the game and the process of habit formation involve avoiding obstacles and accomplishing an objective by using focus and strategy.

Triggers are the stimuli in the environment that lead you to engage in a particular behavior. The behavior that predictably, or regularly, follows a trigger is the **action**. You repeat the action over and over to experience the perceived benefit, or **gain**.

Rachel, for example, used the power of the habit loop to develop a habit of getting 8 hours of sleep per night.

She set an alarm for 10:30 p.m. to build in a reminder that it was time to turn off the television and prepare for bed. The alarm (trigger) signaled that it was time to engage in her bedtime ritual (action) which led her to go to sleep by 11:00 p.m. each night. After practicing this for several weeks, she had created a new habit loop that led her to feel more rested and calmer during the day (gain).

This book will help you become better at understanding your own habit loops, and will also help you use the power of habit loops to develop positive habits and crush bad habits. For each habit described in the chapters that follow, I have suggested a gain that you might experience, such as noticing your mood lift after trying a new self-care behavior. You may not be accustomed to paying such close attention to your reactions, so this is to provide you with options rather than to describe how you will feel.

What's Happening in the Brain

What happens externally when a habit forms is only the tip of the iceberg. Scientists are still trying to get the full picture of what happens in the brain when habits form and whether the process is the same across populations. Dr. Ann Graybiel, a professor at MIT, and her colleague revealed in a 2015 study that a structure in the brain, the dorsolateral striatum, is activated during the habit formation process.

The first time you engage in a behavior, activity in the dorsolateral striatum is set off. When you repeat that behavior enough times, the associated behaviors are chunked together by your brain.

High-stress situations are most compelling for the brain, meaning that habits are formed more strongly under stressful conditions. A signal occurs in the brain at the start of the behavior and again upon the last behavior that routinely occurs in the series, bookending the chunked behaviors at the start *and* end of the behavioral chain. The aforementioned study's research posits that the brain has difficulty moving to a new behavior until the current behavior chain is completed. This theory suggests that what locks in habits is the brain's strong urge to carry out learned patterns of behavior and that it resists subsequent tasks when a pattern diverges from its expectations. For example, if you don't engage in your regular 15-minute walk at 3:00 p.m., your brain signals your body that something is amiss, and you may have difficulty focusing on your work afterward.

It is important to understand that building and breaking habits is not just about willpower. Instead, there are brain-based physiological reasons that support the process of maintaining habits. Armed with this knowledge, you can better navigate the habit formation process, its ups and downs, and particularly how it relates to bad habits.

What about Bad Habits?

Over the years, my coaching and therapy clients have come to me because they wanted to feel better and live in a more relaxed and happy way. Most often, this has required looking at behaviors and habits that do not serve their highest vision for their lives. To help them shed light on the changes they need to make, we look at the impact of the bad habit.

To understand how bad habits work, let's examine a common example. Imagine you're a child who is having an experience that is causing a stressful reaction (trigger). To calm you, your parents give you a piece of chocolate (action). The chocolate tastes good and causes you to calm down (i.e., it provides a short-term gain but doesn't actually resolve the trigger). Over time, you establish the habit of eating chocolate to calm yourself down in stressful situations. Although it does so momentarily, your mind and body are still feeing stress from the unresolved situation, and eventually that creates wear and tear on the body.

On a physiological level, bad habits are developed and maintained when the gain activates reward centers in the brain. Often, the development of bad habits is encouraged by short-term gains that, like the chocolate in the example, don't truly address the trigger. Over time, these bad habits masking the trigger can have a negative impact on one's well-being, daily functioning, relationships, educational goals, or professional life.

Bad habits don't just happen in a vacuum; they happen in a larger environmental or cultural context that is influenced by a person's microsystem (family, friends, social groups) and macrosystem (media, educational systems, institutions). Modern living provides a barrage of environmental stimuli and offers us models for how we ought to behave, consume, or buy. Bad habits often occur as a way to accommodate the world and the overwhelming 24/7 stimuli it brings—which coincidentally goes against our true nature. Although we may live in modern times, our bodies are still programmed to thrive in simpler environments.

Remember, bad habits initially form out of an unconscious desire to help ourselves. But your energy is often focused on mitigating stress rather than truly nurturing yourself. The discomfort associated with your bad habits contributes to your overall level of stress and well-being, because the longer a trigger goes without being addressed, the greater negative impact it has on your sense of joy, your fulfillment in life, and your happiness in your relationships.

Bad Habit Loop

Recall that habits are developed when you associate a certain cue with a specific action, the reward of which encourages the brain to repeat it. With enough repetition, the associated behaviors chunk together to become a habit that is then automatized. The automatic behavior resumes each time the brain recognizes the trigger, which instigates a chain of actions so the brain can experience the gain associated with it. When this automated behavior, or habit, detracts from your overall well-being, or your personal, educational, or professional life, you've gotten caught up in the bad habit loop.

Habit loops, especially around bad habits, are particularly impacted by context. Often, a habit that was adaptive, or made sense for your life when first developed, no longer makes sense within the circumstances of your current life. Take, for example, Courtney's college habit of starting to work on essays and papers the night before they were due to accommodate the two part-time jobs that were funding their associate degree. Back then, the strategy made sense, because they could turn out a paper that received high marks even under strict time constraints.

Let's break Courtney's habit loop down. Receiving an assignment (trigger) led to writing it with limited time (action), which led to high grades and the adrenaline rush of getting work done at the last minute (gain). Of course Courtney would continue this behavior.

Later in life, as a manager responsible for writing complex quarterly sales reports, Courtney starts the projects the night before they are due. Waiting until the last minute has led Courtney to feel overwhelmed and in a constant state of dread over completing the deliverable. The behavior continues because the final product is always well received, but stress of the process outweighs the perceived gain.

The process for breaking bad habits provides clues about how Courtney can get out of this situation. When moving away from bad self-care habits to ones that have a more positive impact on your life, the gain associated with the new, healthier behavior is initially going to be less compelling. But with repetition, the gain will deepen; therefore, for each new habit in the pages that follow, I will guide you to notice the gain for each habit.

Breaking Bad Habits

Bad habits are developed slowly over time and become so automatic that it's easy to mistake the behaviors for part of your personality, thinking that's just the way you are. It's equally easy to forget that there was a time when the habit did not exist. For example, you may have learned the habit as a child before your brain was fully developed or before you even had language. Take, for instance, a person who grew up in a volatile household and saw their parents erupt in anger during moments of stress. It would come as no surprise that the same person developed a habit of yelling at their partner during tense moments.

Changing bad habits requires conscious attention and curiosity regarding the behavior over a sustained period of time. In 2010, researchers at Duke University announced they had found that people need to "vigilantly monitor" bad habits they want to change. Vigilant monitoring allows people an opportunity to use the planning and processing centers of the brain to inhibit the urge to engage in the bad habit and to instead practice a new, more positive habit. But let's be honest—that type of self-monitoring is challenging in the 21st century, so it must be learned.

A different option is to remove yourself from environmental triggers altogether. However, most of us can't actually leave to correct a habit that negatively impacts our life. But what one can pay attention to, and what this book highlights, is how to create new environmental triggers to engage with to replace bad habits. I've applied this principle to my work with all types of clients by helping them look at the environmental triggers to their bad habits.

Although it is hard to break bad habits, it is not impossible! In order to be successful, it's important to have a realistic understanding of the challenges associated with changing bad habits and to develop a plan that will help you overcome those challenges.

Self-Care Habits

Let's begin with an exercise.

Take out a sheet of paper and create two columns. On the left, list the new habits you've hoped to establish for years but haven't quite gotten around to. On the right, list the bad habits you would like to change. What you likely notice while looking at the list is a couple of things. First, it is rather stressful to carry the emotional weight of not living in a way that you know intuitively would feel better. Second, if you are like many of my clients, you are feeling surprised at how such little things impact the way you feel about yourself.

You don't have to feel this way! Here's where self-care comes in:

You *can* go from spending most of your daily free time on social media and isolating from others to balancing social media with time connecting with friends, walking in nature, or journaling.

You *can* make healthier meal choices.

You *can* feel more relaxed on a daily basis.

Augustine, a busy second-year law student, was able to go from being adamantly opposed to self-care, viewing it as a time suck, to someone who created a daily schedule that included at least three self-care habits. He even gave a workshop about the importance of self-care at the next new student orientation, to equip first-year law students with this knowledge.

The following chapters will provide you with easy and practical strategies to enhance your self-care.

KEY TAKEAWAYS

- Habits form consciously and unconsciously. After repeated occurrences, the behaviors associated with your habits get linked together, become automatic, and are strengthened in your brain.

- Habits formed under stressful circumstances can be the most challenging to change.

- Although there are behavioral and biological reasons that make it difficult to change habits, it is possible to do so, especially when you are aware of the TAG (Trigger, Action, Gain) process, you have a plan, and you use proven techniques to overcome challenges.

- Changing your bad habits and developing new, healthier habits puts you on a path to increased self-care, which can benefit your overall well-being.

How to Build Better Self-Care Habits

When you begin to build healthier habits, you also enhance your self-care. In doing so, you build a set of powerful strategies that you can draw from throughout the course of your life. After reading chapter 2, you will better understand the power of self-care, how to develop self-care habits, and how to replace bad habits. You will also gain insight into how small habit changes, added together over the course of time, can change your life for the better. All of this will help ground your awareness in some of the most effective strategies available to support habit change.

Improve Self-Care, Transform Your Life

Self-care is an essential strategy for replenishing oneself from the daily onslaught of stress. Stress is a normal part of life. The vast access to stimuli that modern life offers has made life easier, but at the same time, it can be overwhelming if left unchecked. Also, given the pace of modern life, it is easy not to have time to be fully at rest and give your body and mind time for recovery.

Keep in mind that, even right now, you are not just dealing with the impact of what happened today or earlier this week but also in the months and even years leading up to today. Nor are you reacting only to your personal experience but rather to what is happening in your family, your community, and in the larger world. All of the stress associated with those processes accumulates and contributes to what has been termed "allostatic load": the accumulation of unresolved stress over the course of a lifetime. This can lead to emotional and physical "weathering," especially for people who hold marginalized identities.

My favorite definition of self-care comes from a nursing researcher, Dorothea Orem, who describes self-care as "the practice of activities that individuals initiate and perform on their own behalf in maintaining life, health, and well-being." The benefit of engaging in regular self-care habits is that it builds resilience, or the ability to navigate stressful times. Positive psychology theory offers that it is helpful to consider well-being habits as worthwhile for their own sake, with enhanced happiness and life satisfaction as by-products. Engaging in self-care also has many wellness benefits, including making your life better overall through increased self-esteem and a positive outlook.

When an individual engages in self-care exercises, they are often able to be healthier in their relationships: less irritated when a direct report at work makes a mistake, more able to receive feedback from their partner, more vibrant overall, and better able to rebound when difficulties arise. I've also seen, as well-being theory posits, that well-being is bidirectional. That means that when one member of a family or community models self-care, it benefits other members of the community as well, starting a domino effect.

You might have noticed that I have not described self-care in terms of buying products, services, or equipment or taking trips, because those benefits are temporary. All of those things can be fun, and I encourage you to engage in episodic self-care gestures when it works for you and to the extent that they fit into your budget. Instead, I encourage you to consider how to build long-term self-care habits that you can turn to at any time. In the chapters ahead, I will teach you easy ways to incorporate self-care habits into your everyday life.

Keep in mind that self-care is not a cure-all, nor is it a substitute for mental health or medical treatment. Rather, self-care is an adjunct to professional services and a preventive measure for health issues that are not biologically based. Self-care is about what you do on a regular basis to demonstrate the way you value yourself and your well-being. Taking care of yourself doesn't require having tons of money or time, and it isn't dependent upon your social status. Since there's no one-size-fits-all approach, you can customize a plan for self-care habits that fits your preference and life context.

Develop Your Self-Care Habits

As you start out on your journey to actively improve your self-care habits, it's important to assess your current situation with open eyes. You cannot change what you are not aware of. With that in mind, think first about the healthy habits you currently possess and how they make your life easier and more enjoyable. Applaud yourself for the self-care–enhancing habits you currently have. Now observe any of your bad habits with curiosity rather than judgment. Remind yourself that you can create new habits and release counterproductive ones to increase your self-care. Recognize that your self-care is a work in progress and that, with the help of this book, you will use science and best practices to develop new self-care habits.

As you bring conscious attention to the current state of your self-care, it is helpful to be clear about what factors in your life keep you from taking better care of yourself. Take an inventory of your daily habits: Ask yourself honestly, are they contributing to your well-being, or are they things you have been doing because you have always been doing them? Are you marathon-watching the latest streaming series late into the night because everyone else is talking about it? Are you working from home all day, at night, and on weekends? Is the kids' time taking up all of your time? What you're looking for is an optimal balance between what you give to yourself, what you give to other people, and what you give to the tasks and responsibilities in your life. The degree of harmony among these aspects of life will be different for each person.

You can develop new habits for self-care rather easily, but for them to become automatic, it does take a time commitment. I like to describe self-care habits as a daily multivitamin for your well-being. Like vitamins, you don't take them for immediate benefits or as a magic cure. Instead, you take them as a way to replenish your body with sustenance that you wouldn't otherwise get without conscious attention. It can take an estimated 59 to 66 days for a new habit to become automatic. The information in the latter chapters will guide you through that process. Don't think of this as daunting but rather as clarifying motivation enabling you to commit to giving yourself time for the new self-care habit that will become ingrained.

We will focus on 10 key areas in the chapters to come. They are as follows:

1. Physical activity in fun and easy ways
2. Eating habits that nourish you
3. Connecting with others meaningfully
4. Creating better conditions to sleep well
5. Taking breaks to increase overall relaxation
6. Self-compassion to be gentler with yourself
7. Supporting your brain to aid in its functioning

8. Stress management to learn how to reduce stress
9. Spending time outdoors to connect with the healing benefits of nature
10. Mindfulness to bring conscious attention to living in the moment

Small Changes, Big Results

In this book, you'll learn the research-based, time-tested, and practice-informed strategies that I teach my clients to help you make changes and gain the results you desire. You'll start with mindset and thinking big (i.e., "I *can* change"). Then you'll need to set a clear goal and couple it with bite-size goals, or habits, that will help you achieve it. You'll find that simple changes added together lead to significant and meaningful results. Each small habit that you develop becomes hardwired in the brain, which leads the behavior to become automatic when you encounter its associated trigger.

Developing a goal is the foundation of the change process. Before creating a goal, it is helpful to identify your compelling reason (your big *why*) for making changes in your life. You've read several reasons for self-care and the associated benefits, and you picked up this book for a reason. What is that reason? What is that thing that has told your heart and mind that you want better self-care habits overall? Take a moment to think of your answer and write it down. Here are some examples of a big why:

Example A: I want to have more energy so that I enjoy life outside of work.

Example B: I want to develop healthy habits that I can pass on to my children.

Example C: I want to have more joy in my life so that I can feel more comfortable connecting with others.

When developing your goal, create it in the SMART goal format. SMART stands for Specific, Measurable, Attainable, Realistic, and Time-bound. So, rather than setting a generic goal that you want to be healthier, start with one component of health, like physical activity, and write a SMART goal, such as: *By November 8, I will be able to jog two miles without becoming winded.*

To achieve your overall goal, you will develop habits. Here are some of the core strategies and concepts that will be used in this book to address your habits.

→ **Habit stacking:** adding a new habit onto an already ingrained habit.

→ **Vigilant monitoring:** monitoring your behaviors and cravings and saying to yourself, "Don't do it," to counteract the urge to engage in a bad habit.

→ **Pairing and praise:** coupling tiny, easy changes with a regular activity and engaging in self-praise.

→ **Creating efficiencies:** streamlining your routine to counteract decision fatigue.

→ **Environmental change:** altering the environment to avoid triggers.

→ **Habit substitution:** finding a healthier alternative to a current habit.

For extra credit, before moving on to the next chapter, I recommend that you get five index cards and label them *My Why, Benefits, Drawbacks, Obstacles and Solutions* and *My New Life*. (In case you are wondering why you are listing drawbacks in regard to your goal, there is always a perceived downside to change, and we want to call that out so you can assess whether the benefits outweigh the perceived negative aspects.) Write the answers to those prompts on the respective cards and read the cards a few times a day. Doing so can help you counteract "future discounting," or the tendency to minimize the future benefits of changes in the present, and plan for how you'll deal with challenges along the way.

KEY TAKEAWAYS

- Self-care habits are behaviors that support your overall well-being, often with the happy side effect of increased happiness and positive emotions.

- Awareness of your current level of self-care is important. You cannot change what you do not know, but it is important to be curious and honest rather than judge yourself.

- Building new self-care habits and releasing bad habits is best accomplished using effective, research-informed strategies. There is no one-size-fits-all plan to self-care. The best self-care plan is one that includes habits that endure. It can take up to 66 days to make a new habit automatic, so make sure not to give up prematurely.

- Developing and demonstrating self-care habits in your home, at work, and in your community has the additional benefit of promoting well-being and self-care in others.

- Complete the activities suggested throughout chapter 2, as they help support the change process.

BUILDING HEALTHY SELF-CARE HABITS

Now that you have an understanding of the habit formation process, you'll learn how to apply it. The chapters ahead offer internal self-care, like practicing self-compassion, and external, like increasing physical activity.

You can read the chapters sequentially or start with any chapter from part 2 that calls to you. Remember to use your habit trackers and give yourself adequate time to develop the habit rather than stopping before the habit sticks.

CHAPTER 3

Getting Physical

T his chapter covers how to develop healthy physical activity and exercise habits to cultivate self-care. Remember gym class growing up and all of the joys and sorrows associated with it? Though it may not have always been fun, the best thing about institutionalized exercise is that it creates a habit. When circumstances change, new habits, like bringing in more exercise and physical activity, need to be formed for positive self-care. The habits in this chapter focus on integrating movement into your everyday life. Please remember to check with your doctor before introducing any new forms of exercise.

Why Physical Activity Matters

Regular exercise has several benefits that most of us are aware of: it improves sleep quality, mood, and cognitive performance; it helps prevent or manage health conditions such as cancer, diabetes, and high blood pressure, and it helps with depression as an important adjunct to medication. Yet many people find it challenging to make time for physical activity.

In my experience over two decades of working with all types of people, at all fitness levels, one of the most compelling but infrequently considered reasons for exercise is that it's one of the best ways to mitigate stress and brings the body to a place of recovery after a difficult period. I believe that those who shift their mindset about exercising to focus on this reason are likely to take it up.

In future chapters, I'll go into more depth about the role that stress plays in the body, but for now, ground your awareness in an understanding: when you experience stress, your body has a physiological response, and it is best served by periods of recovery after that stress. Physical activity helps with that. So you can dance for 20 minutes at the end of your day, take an exercise class at lunch, or do some in-home calisthenics. The goal is to integrate physical activity habits into your life so that you can come down from stress—and reap all of the other benefits of exercise in the process.

Building Healthier Habits

It is clear that exercise has important benefits for people who regularly engage in it. Unless your physician has told you otherwise, there is very little reason to avoid exercise. As you can imagine, it's likely that the lack of exercise is related to the absence of physical activity habits. In this chapter we will focus on ways that you can add more physical activity to things you do on a regular basis and cultivate specific habits to help you increase movement in your life.

Moving forward, try to shift your mindset (if it's not already there) to think about physical activity as a part of what you do every day—not confining it to what we typically think of as exercise, nor requiring a gym.

So before you begin, take some deep breaths. Acknowledge your feelings—perhaps trepidation, or even resistance to exercise. Let go of your judgment about times when you tried to exercise and then gave up, or the fact that you are not in the same shape you used to be. Instead, turn inward to ask if there is a bit of excitement or curiosity that you might be willing to turn up. From that space, no matter how tiny, jump into the habits below.

Jazz Up Household Chores

This first habit may be surprisingly easy to develop, because it's simply powering up what may be a preexisting routine: household chores. Housework burns calories and gets your heart rate up. Vacuuming is exercise (119 calories per 60 minutes), just like sweeping the floors (136 calories per 30 minutes), cleaning the tub (90 calories per 15 minutes), and washing the car (153 calories per 30 minutes). AND you can add to the benefit of these activities by embellishing them—adding a little flourish or a bit more vigor. For example, move your feet while cleaning your countertop, do some calf raises while dusting a shelf, take a longer route to the trash receptacle when taking out the trash, or stand and do toe taps while decluttering your cabinets.

1. Pick a set of chores that you do regularly each week. The chore is the trigger for the upcoming action.
2. Plan a strategy for embellishing your chores by moving another part of your body while doing it.
3. Do your housework for at least 5 minutes and work up to 15 minutes over time to get maximum benefit.

Not only will you support your exercise goals and derive the physical benefits from this habit, but you'll also have the additional benefit of a consistently clean and clutter-free home.

Helpful Tip:
→ If you would like to add a bit more movement to your household tasks, consider adding some traditional exercises, like squats, at the beginning or end of your task, or both.

Walk More in Daily Life

Humans are meant to move and be active, but our lives are often sedentary. Even if you already take an exercise class or belong to a gym, your body and mind will thank you if you make it a habit to incorporate moments of rejuvenating activity throughout your day.

List your 10 most common passive habits, such as emailing colleagues who are a short walk away from your cubicle or texting family members when you are in the same home. Brainstorm a tiny step you can take to make the habit more active. Start with the first three items on your list.

1. When you encounter any of the items on your list, make the transition from being passive to active. For example, when you reach for your phone to text a family member who is downstairs, tell yourself, "Don't do it," then walk downstairs instead.

2. Congratulate yourself every time you successfully engage in your new habit.

By incorporating more activity throughout your day, you may notice that you gradually gain a sense of vitality and an increased ability to manage or recover from daily stressors.

Helpful Tips:

→ After the first three habits are ingrained, start working on the next three habits (or however many you can reasonably take on and still be successful). Before you know it, your sedentary life will be a thing of the past!

→ For an extra challenge, when you would normally take an elevator or escalator, try taking the stairs instead—even if you only walk up one flight and take an elevator the rest of the way.

Get Up and Dance

This dance break habit builds on your association between music and movement. Many people have a few songs that make them want to get up and dance. Choose one or two of these tracks each morning and dance to them for 3 to 5 minutes, then gradually work your way up to five or six tracks and 15 to 20 minutes. To start, create a playlist of five to ten songs you love to dance to and set them to shuffle on your device. Shuffling the songs provides some variety from day to day and prevents boredom.

1. Pick a date on your calendar to begin your new routine and determine what regular activity you will pair it with. (Remember, habit stacking with an already ingrained habit can make the adoption of new habits easier.) For example, you might decide to begin dancing while brushing your teeth or just afterward.

2. When you push play and hear the first song, get up and dance.

Savor how the sounds and rhythms move through your body and embrace the elevated mood that the music and movement bring you.

Helpful Tips:

→ If you have a limited range of movement or you move with the assistance of a mobility device, remain seated, let your mind engage with the music, and move to the extent that you are able.

→ If you prefer pairing this with an evening activity, make it an evening cooldown and dance to music that helps you wind down. Just make sure you don't do it too close to bedtime.

Wake Up and Work Out

The best form of exercise is the one that you will actually do. So with this habit, it's less important to choose the most efficacious forms of exercise and more important to choose a small group of exercises that feel good to you and engage your body on a regular basis. This habit is especially helpful if you currently do not engage in any exercise.

Pick five to seven exercises that you would like to commit to doing daily. Examples include sit-ups, squats, jumping jacks, push-ups, leg lifts, or arm raises. You can easily search YouTube for sample exercises by entering keywords that meet your needs, such as "chair exercise," "exercises for beginners," and so on.

1. Upon waking, complete five reps (repetitions) of each of the exercises in your set. Do the exercises in the same order each day.

2. As the habit becomes ingrained, gradually add reps (one rep each time you work out, or five reps each week—whatever you can manage safely without over-doing it) until you can do two sets of ten reps of each of your chosen exercises.

Appreciate how invigorated your body feels.

→ Over time, if you find yourself becoming bored or overusing particular muscles, you'll want to vary your main set of exercises by adding new ones or focusing on different muscle groups on different days.

→ While 30 minutes of physical activity a day is optimal, this habit coupled with one of the others in this chapter is a great place to start.

Breaking Bad Habits

Many people don't like exercise, so they simply don't do it. Since exercise is the easiest way to complete the stress cycle, its importance cannot be understated. To overcome nonexistent, inconsistent, or unhealthy exercise habits, you'll want to uncover the beliefs and biases you have about exercise. Next, look at the barriers that you currently face concerning exercise.

When you think about the images of people that you see on television, on your computer screen, and in magazines, it's likely that you notice that there's a fairly singular pattern and aesthetic of what happy, healthy, and beautiful bodies look like. The media's message is that exercise is for someone thin, flexible, younger, or already fit.

In reality, the average body size of an American woman is larger than most of the images that appear in the media. Your body deserves physical activity whatever its size. Exercise for the purposes of reducing stress and maintaining health is positive for anyone at any age and of every ability type. If you pay attention to who you are and ignore the media's voice about who you should be, you are more likely to take better care of yourself.

Failing to Make Time

A key reason people do not exercise is because they have made an unrealistic appraisal of their schedule and therefore have not identified a dedicated time for exercise. When you pick a regular day and time and stick to it repeatedly, over time your body will begin to crave that movement and prepare to engage in it as scheduled.

I will never forget the aha moment I had while listening to a panel of college presidents during a leadership training program. Each panelist mentioned waking up early each day to engage in some form of exercise. Busy as they were, they made time for exercise.

1. Find a time in your calendar when you can reliably exercise without interruption.
2. Schedule a recurring weekly appointment with a reminder at that time.

Helpful Tips (choose one that will keep you accountable and that makes the most sense for you):

→ Attend a regular fitness class with an instructor or classmates you enjoy. You'll get the physical benefits as well as the social connection.

→ Hire a trainer. Paying for a service makes you *far* more likely to show up for it.

→ Enlist a walking buddy. A companion who you don't want to let down will help keep you accountable.

→ Join a free fitness group and make friends. Social influence cannot be downplayed.

→ Search YouTube for videos with instructors you like. Schedule the workout at a time when you have the least interruptions.

Parking Close to the Door

When I moved from New York City back to the suburbs, where I had spent most of my life, I found myself schooling my city-bred husband in the ways of suburbanites—for instance, when driving to a store even just a few blocks from our house, the goal was to park as close as possible to the door and walk as little as possible. If you recognize yourself in this anecdote, try to replace this habit with a healthier habit that helps you be more active.

1. Think about ways to use your body first, whether that means walking (or, if need be, driving, parking farther away, and walking) or biking to your destination whenever you have to go somewhere close to home.

2. To start, pick one destination and decide how you would like to get there. Test out the route, and if it works for you, elect to use that mode of transportation to get to that destination.

3. Once you have developed this habit, pick another set of locations a little bit farther away. Aim to eventually have at least five places that you walk or bike to on a regular basis.

→ Make sure you walk at times and in locations where it is safe for you to do so.

→ If you are a suburbanite, brace yourself for questions and stares from neighbors!

Sitting All Day

Several years ago, the news media began to describe sitting as the new smoking, with the implication being that this seemingly harmless activity actually has immense health consequences. If you are an office worker, you may feel exhausted at the end of a long day of sitting. So when you get home, you spend the rest of the evening "relaxing" in a seated position.

Sitting too much can negatively impact your mood, put you at risk for illness and body discomfort, and even negate the progress you have made from exercising. Therefore, it's important to get up out of your seat multiple times a day.

1. At the start of the week, plan to work in 60-minute chunks. Set a timer to help keep you on track.

2. Stand for five minutes and, if possible, walk around your work space before returning to your desk.

3. Repeat this cycle throughout the day. Notice how much better your body feels each time you sit back down.

→ If you have medical reasons for sitting throughout the day, check with your physician to see if tensing muscles through progressive muscle relaxation is an appropriate replacement activity.

→ If you stand for work, quicken your pace or add in a couple of quick and easy exercises when you walk to the restroom or on other breaks to mix things up.

Tracking Your Progress

Use this tracker as a tool to help you monitor your progress and gain insight into why a habit perhaps isn't quite sticking. We track our habits so we can learn, modify, and improve.

HABIT	M	T	W	TH	F	SAT	S

KEY TAKEAWAYS

- Focus on giving your body an experience that has not only physical but also health and mood-enhancing benefits.

- Physical activity is the best way to complete the stress cycle. It lets your body know it can unwind after the stresses of the day. Focusing on the stress-relieving benefits can help you commit, especially if the physical benefits are not sufficiently compelling for you.

- The best exercise is the one you do consistently. Have a few go-to exercises and a regular time to perform them to habituate physical activity.

- Social incentive will give you a boost. Scheduling some form of group or paired exercise is a helpful way to get started with habits you're not enthusiastic about.

CHAPTER 4

Eating Better

What distinguishes good from bad eating habits? When you incorporate TAG (see page 5) into your understanding of eating habits, it is important to pay attention to the triggers for your eating, the actions that you take to eat, and, particularly, the gains you are striving to make. Good eating habits take your goal of self-care into account, whereas bad habits are breakdowns of your triggers, redirections of your actions, and distractions from your goal—all of which can leave you feeling unfulfilled. In this chapter, I will discuss four different habits that contribute to healthy eating and then touch on three common bad habits related to our eating practices. Please know that if you experience disordered eating or are in recovery, you should rely on the advice of your healthcare professionals before engaging in any of these habits.

Why Healthy Eating Matters

You would think that eating is the simplest thing in the world, and it is, but eating *well* can be quite complicated to do. When you are a very young child, you are guided by the wisdom of the body. Your internal bodily cues help you understand when you're hungry and when you're full. You are guided toward healthy food choices even before you consciously know what that means.

In childhood, you begin to be more influenced by your parents, peers, media, and environment. Then, as you grow and develop, especially from adolescence and adulthood, eating becomes influenced by cultural and social phenomena. With all of these distractions, it's easy to allow the external to take precedence over the internal and to become disconnected from that accurate, once-trusted bodily wisdom of your very early life. When your eating habits become particularly reliant upon the norms you see in your environment, *your* priorities can get pushed aside and misplaced.

Healthy eating supports cell growth and regeneration, delivers the energy the body needs to maintain bodily systems and perform daily tasks, and even provides pleasure. Professionals recommend focusing your attention back on your body's wisdom; the more you listen to what your body needs, the less you are influenced by external messaging.

Building Healthier Habits

The most effective eating habits incorporate the wisdom of your body and balance it with the demands placed on you as you navigate living in an ever-changing environment. This wisdom guides your body's food-related priorities, such as using food as fuel and as a way to bolster the immune system. It also helps you manage the external cues that encourage an outsize focus on eating pleasure.

Now, don't get me wrong, humans are evolutionarily predisposed to eat for pleasure: fatty foods, sugar, salt, and even a degree of gluttony kept our ancestors alive for centuries when food was hard to come by, and those preferences helped them survive tough times. But that's not the world we live in now. Today, there is a whole culture built around consumption, with 24/7 advertising aimed at tempting our taste buds. Thus, it's more important than ever to consciously nurture the predispositions derived from the wisdom of your body and turn them into lifelong habits.

Eat Whole Foods

Your body operates best on whole foods, or foods that are as close to their natural state as possible. So stick with minimally processed proteins and fresh fruit and vegetables. Danish consumer behavior researcher Liliya Nureeva found that adolescents who ate fruits and vegetables had higher self-control when eating. This is likely also true for adults. Although processed foods taste good, they also overstimulate your senses, making you want to eat more because they trigger cravings for sugar, fats, and salt, often by using artificial ingredients.

List five processed foods that you eat regularly. Pick one food with an easy homemade replacement. For example, homemade sweet potato fries are easy to make and require few ingredients, most of which are probably in your cupboard right now. Create a monthly habit of making this item at home instead of having fast-food fries.

1. Set a reminder in your calendar to trigger you to make your chosen food item.

2. Follow your recipe. Where possible, make ahead or double the recipe so that you have a grab-and-go version.

3. Once you have developed a routine with the first food, move to the next food on your list.

Take stock of your increased energy level and satiety level after eating the healthier version.

Helpful Tips:

→ Be patient. When you eat food without additives, give it some time. Your taste buds will need time to adjust to the natural flavor, but when they do, you will never want to go back.

→ If you start children on the healthier homemade version, they will likely prefer it and won't know what they are missing.

Savor Your Food

Let's face it—in this fast-paced world, many meals end up being eaten on the go. When you eat too fast, you rob yourself of the opportunity to appreciate what you're eating. A more relaxed pace allows you to register feelings of fullness and to be more aware of your intake. Eating more mindfully counteracts the impact of stress and the urge to engage in unhealthy eating behaviors.

To start, pick one meal a week to make a full sensory experience. The plan is to make this meal a joyous event. Take the time to set the table, and maybe even create a mood with flowers or a candle on the table.

1. Before you begin eating, breathe in the aroma of the food and pause to take in the appeal of the food on your plate.
2. Eat deliberately.
3. Savor the flavors and textures of your food as you eat.
4. Do this for a week. In each week that follows, add another slow meal to your routine.

Notice how eating in this relaxed state allows you to enjoy your food more fully.

Helpful Tips:

→ Turn off the TV and other forms of entertainment, except music.

→ Buy and eat the best-quality food you can afford. You will often find that you need less to feel satisfied.

Go on a Culinary Tour

Eating a variety of food is an important step to improving your eating habits. When you eat the same meals week after week, you will eventually become bored. Furthermore, stocking your kitchen with the same options all the time can lead to making impulsive food choices for the sake of variety, and impulsive eating can lead to over-indulging in unhealthy, temporarily satisfying foods. You can avoid this meal fatigue by committing to trying new foods, diversifying your diet, and satisfying your taste buds with new flavors.

An easy way to do this is to begin to explore the flavors, spices, and cuisines of other cultures. Pick a day of the week when you will try a new dish. Consider which day of the week you tend to eat your least favorite meal or the day when you have the most time to experiment. Once you pick the day, you can give it a theme, such as "Meatless Mondays," where you try new vegetarian dishes.

1. On the appointed day, make the meal that you researched.

2. Mentally note the flavor combination or texture you most enjoy.

Increasing the variety in your meals and cooking them on your own will lead you to experience the benefits of healthy eating, which can increase your overall feeling of well-being.

Helpful Tips:
→ Prepping is key. Plan a week at a time and pick meals that have similar ingredients.

→ A way to make this habit extra healthy is to find new ways to prepare vegetable dishes in order to help increase your vegetable intake.

→ Make the experience more fun by listening to music from the country or region where the dish originated.

Trust Your Body

In this habit, you will learn how to better understand your body's signal for hunger and its signal for satiety. As you build this habit, use a rating scale to assign a number to your level of fullness and hunger level. At lunch, eat as you normally would until you are full. Rate this as a 10 on your fullness scale of 1 (hungry) to 10 (full). This is your fullness limit. On the following day, wait until you feel hungry rather than eating your midday meal based on a schedule. Just before eating, use the same scale of 1 (hungry) to 10 (full) to notice what hunger feels like. This is your hunger baseline.

1. Eat lunch every day just before you reach the hungry feeling you recorded as your hunger baseline.
2. Check in two times during the meal to give yourself a fullness rating.
3. Stop eating just before you feel full, based on your fullness limit.

As you gain a deeper understanding of your body's signals, you may find that you are less irritable before meals and less sluggish afterward, which may result in an increased sense of overall well-being.

→ Be sure to check with your physician before developing this habit if you experience disordered eating, or to make sure there are no contraindications for only eating when hungry.

→ Either adopt a mindset that you don't have to eat everything on your plate or opt for smaller portions. You can always have a bit more if needed.

Breaking Bad Habits

Eating is contextual, meaning it's often connected to what you learned growing up, your culture, and your life circumstances. If you grew up in a household where there was never enough food or your food intake was monitored by others, you likely have some food habits that allow you to be unbounded in how you eat. Or, eating quickly is a habit that you might develop based on the work you do. If you work shifts as a retail salesperson or as a medical professional, you likely have short breaks accompanied by long hours on your feet, moving from place to place. Thus, your fast-paced life is often reflected in how you eat.

It can feel overwhelming to try to change food habits that do not serve us well. It is helpful to pay attention to what triggers these habits and start small when making adjustments in your behaviors. Three bad habits that are worth getting a jump on are drinking sugary drinks, not chewing food thoroughly, and shopping on an empty stomach.

Drinking Sugary Drinks

When I was in my early adolescence, I remember commercials with sports legends drinking a can of pop after a big win at a stadium. The message was clear: winners drink soda. The thing is, soda has no nutritional value, but the advertising resonates on a deeply cultural and habitual level. The truth is that soda contains a highly addictive substance: sugar. There are on average 10 to 12 teaspoons (about ¼ cup) of sugar in one can of soda. Picture how much sugar that *actually* is. Put simply, do not think of soda as a beverage to drink daily or multiple times a day. Think of soda as a dessert, something to drink only on occasion.

Kicking the soda habit relies on two habit-changing strategies: environmental change and habit substitution. Keeping soda out of your home will help you avoid the trigger involved in seeing it, and substituting a healthy carbonated beverage for soda provides a lightly fruity flavor and the familiar bubbly quality without the added sugar.

1. Remove all of the soda from your home to change the environment.

2. Purchase flavored seltzer water as a substitute for soda.

3. After a month, maintain your flavored seltzer substitution during non-mealtimes, and just drink plain, uncarbonated water around mealtimes.

Helpful Tip:
→ If you cannot do without soda, only drink it when you're out and make your home a soda-free zone.

Not Chewing Food Thoroughly

Digestion, food absorption, and overall gastrointestinal function are all negatively impacted by swallowing food that has not been broken down enough. In addition, not chewing your food fully makes it harder for the body to recognize satiety. Eating slowly and chewing thoroughly ensures that you eat only what you need to be full and prevents overeating.

For this habit, your goal is to chew solid foods for 30 seconds and softer foods for 15 seconds. The strategy that is necessary for the habit change to be successful is vigilant monitoring (as a start, it's helpful to use the timer on your phone or purchase 30- and 15-second sand timers), but over time, when you have developed the habit, your internal timer will tell you roughly how long and how much to chew without an external prompt.

1. For a week, whenever you eat at home, commit to chewing your food for at least 15 or 30 seconds.

2. When you take a bite (or spoonful) of food, use a sand timer and chew until all the sand from the top flows into the lower chamber. It is fine to estimate what halfway looks like if you don't have a 15-second sand timer.

3. Do not pick up your utensils again until you have swallowed your food.

Helpful Tips:

→ It's easy to put too much or too little food in your mouth at one time. Notice what happens when you have chewed for the requisite amount of time. Doing so will help you gauge the size of a reasonable bite. Adjust the next forkful accordingly.

→ This is a helpful habit to build as a couple or family to develop social reinforcement.

Shopping on an Empty Stomach

Having a variety of healthy food choices and limited unhealthy foods on hand at home is an important way to support healthy eating habits. In order to set up your home environment optimally, you'll need to make sure that you shop smart.

There is a lot of time, money, and research that goes into designing a grocery store to entice you to buy processed foods. Consumers often visit grocery stores without a plan to counteract the sophisticated techniques used to trigger emotional purchasing. Shopping when you're hungry will make you especially susceptible to these techniques and is a surefire way to end up with a cart full of products you had no intention of buying before walking in the door.

The most effective strategies for breaking this habit are habit stacking and creating efficiencies. First, stack your weekly shopping trip after a regular meal or snack time, then create efficiencies by shopping on the same day of the week and at the same time every week and always make a list.

1. On your regular shopping day, eat a meal or snack at the usual time, then go to the grocery store.
2. Consult your shopping list and stick to it. If you are tempted to deviate from it, only make healthy selections.
3. Congratulate yourself for shopping smart!

Helpful Tips:

→ If you purchase your groceries online, use the same principles before creating your order. Don't e-shop when hungry!

→ Keep a healthy snack on hand for last-minute or unexpected store runs.

Tracking Your Progress

Use this tracker as a tool to help you monitor your progress and gain insight into why a habit perhaps isn't quite sticking. We track our habits so we can learn, modify, and improve.

HABIT	M	T	W	TH	F	SAT	S

KEY TAKEAWAYS

- Starting new habits like slowing down to savor meals more fully, making small changes that tap into the wisdom of your body, and introducing new foods or preparation methods will set you on a path to healthier eating.

- Using proven strategies to root out your bad habits can help you eat in a way that best serves your body. Some bad habits that you can change right away include drinking sugary drinks, not fully chewing your food, and shopping when you're hungry.

- Always check with your doctor before making any changes in your eating habits.

CHAPTER 5

Staying Connected

Social connections help you meet key psychological needs and help increase life satisfaction. Plus, when you're connecting with others, it helps the people in your life feel the same benefit—it's a win-win situation. To reap the benefits of social connection, you need two important things: variety and authentic connection. This chapter is unique from the others. These habits should be considered more as best practices for developing, strengthening, and nurturing social connections rather than direct interpretations of the TAG system (see page 5).

Why Connecting with Others Matters

The brain experiences social connections in a similar fashion to physical pleasure, delivering a boost of oxytocin, the same neuropeptide that bonds mothers to children and lovers to one another. According to the Greater Good Science Center at UC Berkeley, the quality of your social connections may be the greatest predictor of your well-being.

It is no wonder that noted positive psychology theorist and researcher Martin Seligman's PERMA (Positive emotions, Engagement, Relationships, Meaning, and Accomplishment) model identified relationships as one of the five foundational elements that constitute well-being. The relationship construct highlights the importance your ties to others plays in your life.

Connection is not the mere presence of a relationship, however. It also involves the relationship's quality and depth. Relationships can refer to connections you have with people in your family, social, community, athletic, and religious groups, as well as your coworkers and people who share your hobbies and interests. When you relate authentically with a variety of different people, you create your own unique community. These connections can help you feel happier, live longer, and feel more fulfilled.

Social engagement has benefits throughout life and is particularly helpful as people age. The impact of limited social interaction can be compared to the effects of undue stress, diabetes, and lack of physical activity.

Building Healthier Habits

Given the numerous benefits of healthy social connections, we'll focus on four essential habits that use both
external engagement strategies and internal deepening
strategies for enhancing your relationships.

Your social ties of all types added together form your
personal community. Each relationship within your community has its own meaning and importance. Rather than
focus on relationships that are not quite as connected as
you would hope, focus on the sum total of those social
connections. Starting from that point will allow you to
determine whether to place your energy into deepening
your relationships or into adding variety and enjoyment.

Remember that social connections are an important
part of your self-care. The other chapters of this book
help you strengthen your personal self-care habits, but
this chapter helps you not only improve your own quality
of life but also share the benefits of connection with the
people in your circle and your community.

Deepen Your Existing Relationships

Over the course of your life, you've likely had a friend with
whom you shared a meaningful connection for a certain
length of time, but for whatever reason, you began to see
each other less and less. Then, when you reconnected,
you may have felt like you were picking up right where you
left off. If modern-day life has taken over and made it difficult to maintain meaningful social ties, then you need to
take life back and make that level of depth a priority again.

1. Look through your contact list and write out all the people you haven't spoken to in six months who you used to be in regular contact with.
2. Determine which of these people you would like to reestablish contact with.
3. Text, call, or email someone on your list every day for a week to reestablish contact.
4. In week two, plan to catch up in person with at least one friend.
5. Continue each week thereafter with other people on your list.

Enjoy how regaining contact with old friends enhances your sense of belonging and connection.

Helpful Tips:
→ Pull out your calendar and schedule when you will call friends from past and present. Consider it an appointment.

→ Don't allow yourself to veer off track if people don't respond quickly or at all. Go where the energy is!

→ If people spontaneously pop into your mind to reach out to, just do it!

Join a Hobby or Affiliation Group

Sometimes people do not connect because they feel nervous or awkward about making small talk. Connecting with others through a hobby is particularly helpful for people who are socially shy or anxious, because it provides a shared experience that leads to more organic conversations. What hobby do you practice on your own that you can do with other people? For example, you may love knitting or writing poetry but only do it on your own. Engaging in a related social activity, like joining a knitting or writing group, can be a great way to connect with others.

Check community bulletin boards at your local library or an online listserv to see what groups exist. Often, classes sponsored by your locality, library, or local community college are free or low-cost, so search for those and sign up for them. If there aren't any close to you, then reach out to others you know to see if they would like to set something up with you.

1. Once you've chosen a group or class, clear that time in your schedule and make a commitment to go every week.
2. During each class, make a point of having a conversation with someone else in the class.

You will likely experience the double benefit of enjoying the activity and feeling an increased belonging and connection with others who share your interests.

Helpful Tips:

→ If you go solo and join an established group, allow people time to get to know you and vice versa.

→ Greet people with a smile, a wave, or a hello to signal that you are approachable.

→ Sit with others rather than alone or off to the side.

Volunteer for a Cause You Believe In

Volunteering can become a habit that connects you to like-minded people and creates an ongoing way in which to contribute to your community. You can volunteer with an organization that you already know about (like your religious institution or school alumni association), or you can join a new one. You can also connect with causes that have opportunities for episodic or seasonal volunteer opportunities (like a community farm or local food pantry). Brainstorm a list of causes that you deeply believe in, and if you do not know organizations that already provide this work, do an Internet search for local opportunities to volunteer.

1. Pick one special occasion per quarter when you can give back to others. This can be a holiday, anniversary, or birthday.
2. Contact the organization to schedule.
3. Each time you volunteer, make a point of actively engaging with the people who are there with you.

   In addition to gaining meaningful connections with others in your community when you participate in volunteer activities, you may also enjoy release from stress and an increased sense of purpose.

Helpful Tips:
→ Over the years, my clients who are introverts or have social anxiety have benefitted from starting with periodic volunteer efforts and building up to a more regular, long-standing arrangement over time.

$\rightarrow$ The well-being effects of volunteering can have diminishing returns if you overcommit and do not leave time for yourself to rest. Remember that balance is the key.

Focus on "We" Instead of "Me"

A singular focus on "me" makes any interaction with others simply transactional. In this habit, you will concentrate on broadening your focus. This can be applied to many types of relationships, but the focus here will be on networking, because it reflects the way relationships are often formed in adulthood. Networking is often a transactional interaction in which the goal is seeing what other people can do for "me" in "my" quest for my goal. Many people do, however, develop more meaningful and long-lasting relationships in a business context because they focus on the whole person, which deepens the connection.

1. The next time you are having a networking discussion, pivot and make it a connecting conversation.
2. Ask open-ended questions, like asking the other person to share "the why" about their work rather than just focusing on "the what." Broaden the conversation beyond occupations.
3. Don't interrupt, listen actively and deeply, respond by paraphrasing, and ask follow-up questions.
4. Share your own answers and be yourself.
5. Appreciate what you have learned about the other person.
6. Repeat this habit on a regular basis.

By focusing on "we" instead of "me," you gain an opportunity to deeply know another person and their potential, which can have the added benefit of turning an associate into a friend.

Helpful Tips:

→ At social gatherings, approach one person in a room who at first glance you might not think you have any connection with. This can help widen your social circle.

→ Variety deepens meaning in our lives. If you can, introduce people who you know but do not know each other so that your circle keeps growing.

Breaking Bad Habits

The conditions that make people disconnect from others are often gradual in nature and prompted by external pressures and internal ennui.

On one hand, the modern world can make crushing time demands. Work can be a primary culprit, with people spending more and more time at work, and spending their work time solitarily. Many people eat lunch at their desk alone for only 15 minutes and work all the way through it. But work isn't the only thing that can interfere with your relationships. Social media and electronic games, even idle Internet searching, can become a habit that distracts you from your friends and opportunities to make new acquaintances. Factor in the plethora of cable and streaming programming that you can binge-watch all weekend, and it should come as no surprise that you may have a cluster of habits that takes you away from human contact.

Take stock of the relationships in your life, identify the habits that you'd like to change, and then develop a plan for doing so. Remember, improving your social connections serves you and the people in your life.

Not Making Time for Relationships

A conundrum of modern life is that people who desperately want more connections don't seem to have time to make them. I can't tell you how many times I have had someone tell me how much they want to have more friends and have more fun in their lives but feel unable to make time to meet their goals. Let's face it: developing relationships as an adult requires time, energy, and, of course, interest. As we age, our social circle may get smaller and more intimate; for some, it disappears.

For this habit, your work is to identify the variety of relationships in your life and commit time, like, *actual* time for those relationships. You probably have casual, situational and deep friendships in your life. Each of those relationships is useful and important. Having a broad range of social relationships–from acquaintances to close friends to significant others–is good for your health and professional success.

1. Do a deep dive into your calendar and determine how much time you have for social activity. Aim for 20 percent of your schedule.
2. Block out time for socializing!

3. Contact friends to see in that time.

4. Have fun and cherish the feeling of doing so.

Helpful Tips:

→ When you feel the urge to cancel due to other demands, ask yourself whether it is really necessary to do so.

→ Make plans with a variety of people, including acquaintances.

Maintaining Uneven Relationships

It's necessary to have social connections that are reciprocal, meaning that there is some measure of give-and-take between both parties. Without reciprocity, you develop defined roles in which one person is the giver and the other is the taker. Those kinds of relationships are often more stressful than any benefit they could possibly give.

It's tempting to focus on the person who is asking for more than they actually provide in the relationship in terms of emotional support and connection. What I find more compelling is that those who are on the other side of those relationships are sometimes more comfortable giving and being present to others than allowing themselves to receive. This teaches the receivers in their life that they do not need to give the same level of support. This habit provides a structure for evening out such relationships.

1. Think about the people in your life with whom you have an uneven relationship and determine who is capable of more.

2. Plan a conversation with the person to let them know you are open to receiving more support from them.

3. Ask if they would be willing to explore a reorganization of your roles.

Helpful Tips:

→ For the people on your list who cannot offer a more reciprocal relationship, determine whether it makes sense to calibrate your giving.

→ Focus your emotional energy and expectations on your most satisfying relationships.

Keeping Your Emotional Walls Up

Over the years, one of my specialties has been working with people who, despite their best intentions, have trouble connecting with others. This often has to do with challenging friendships or relational experiences in their past. The truth is, connecting with others is joyful, but it can open you up to misunderstandings and hurt feelings, sometimes leading to distrust. Socially connected people know and accept that possibility; what they don't do is set themselves up for that to be a likely probability.

1. Notice when the urge to put your walls up presents itself.

2. Think, instead, about putting up windows to protect you while letting you see what is out there.

3. If you are comfortable with what you see, then you can open up the windows for more engagement and

confirm that what you see is right for you. Do this by sharing a bit more about your thoughts or feelings than is typical. Notice the reaction.

4. After that, if everything checks out, climb out of the window to really engage.

Helpful Tip:

→ Have an affirmation that you repeat to yourself. For example: "I am a good judge of character, and I can discern who I can let in."

Tracking Your Progress

Use this tracker as a tool to help you monitor your progress and gain insight into why a habit perhaps isn't quite sticking. We track our habits so we can learn, modify, and improve.

HABIT	M	T	W	TH	F	SAT	S

KEY TAKEAWAYS

- Social connection is key to good health and successful aging, so make sure to make time for it.

- Social connections are important for a life well-lived. It is important to allow yourself to have different types of relationships, because you are a person who has many types of needs.

- Given that adulthood comes with responsibilities, you'll need to carve out time to build connections, or they are unlikely to happen.

- It's important to consciously build and nurture your social connections.

CHAPTER 6

Sleeping Better

Sleeping well on a regular basis has numerous benefits. Although there is overwhelming evidence that sleep is essential for physical, emotional, and cognitive function, the fact is that most people do not get enough sleep. Some act as if getting little sleep is a badge of honor. Or it is taken as a given that certain phases of one's life necessitate sleeplessness. In this chapter, we will explore ways to improve the quality of your sleep. I will share with you some common reasons your sleep is impacted, a few of which may surprise you. I will also offer easy-to-implement habits for improving the quality of your sleep and deepening your self-care in this area.

Why Healthy Sleep Matters

In today's culture we are accustomed to living with a sleep deficit. There is an acceptable norm that sleeping well or being well-rested is for vacations or retirement—or even more drastically, the common saying "I will sleep when I'm dead."

Most people don't actually know how much sleep they need. Melinda Beck, a reporter for the *Wall Street Journal*, has noted research that found only 1 to 3 percent of people are able to operate on five to six hours of sleep.

Sleep hygiene refers to the environmental and behavioral strategies one employs to get adequate rest. Your body operates optimally when you complete the four stages of sleep four to six times consecutively. This includes cycling through deep sleep and REM sleep, which allow you to feel well-rested and have energy when you are awake. This chapter focuses on helping you treat sleep as the precious, yet accessible, commodity that it is.

When you are well-rested, your circadian rhythms operate to make you feel better and help you better navigate your daily life.

There are several other benefits of healthy sleep. Good sleep hygiene has been found to support creativity and help job and academic performance. Over the years, I have found helping my clients improve their sleep hygiene can bring about a dramatic change in how they feel and their ability to make other positive changes in their lives. As one client said: "I just feel clearer now that I am sleeping better."

Building Healthier Habits

If you grew up having a bedtime and regular time to rise in the morning, you may have begrudgingly adhered to those household rules. It turns out that there is wisdom in planning the time when you sleep and wake. The body's natural patterns, called circadian rhythms, are synchronized with sunrise and sunset. Having a regular sleep pattern strengthens your body's sleep-wake cycle, stabilizes your circadian rhythms, and supports long-term sleep quality. Most adults need at least seven hours of sleep per night. This practice will help you get the sleep that you need but may not be getting on a regular basis.

To be clear, there can be real barriers to getting adequate sleep. Strengthening your sleep habits can help make a serious dent in these challenges and support your health and well-being overall. I encourage you to pick the habits that best fit your circumstances and commit to trying them for a couple of months. You may be surprised by how effective habituating even one of these behaviors can be!

Create a Receptive Environment for Sleep

Ideally, your bedroom is used only for sleep, intimacy, and recovery from illness, so that the body understands what it is doing when you are using that room. But the reality for many is that a space dedicated to sleep is a luxury. You may not have another location for your desk, your partner may have a strong preference for television in the bedroom, or you may live with others and have limited communal space. Rather than focus on the barriers to having a room just for sleeping, use this habit to optimize your bedroom for sleep by creating a transition plan.

When you enter your bedroom to rest, you want the environment to signal to your body that you are transitioning from waking activities to sleeping. You can do this by making your bedroom your own sleeping oasis.

1. After you put on your pajamas, or about 30 minutes before you go to bed, set the mood for sleep.

2. Reset your bedroom from the tasks of the day, especially if it is used as your office or workstation. Remove your computer from the room or cover it.

3. Adjust the temperature based on what feels right for you. Err on the side of a cooler temperature and adjust your clothing or blankets accordingly.

4. Dim the lights and close the curtains to block outside light.

5. If it helps relax you, sprinkle lavender or chamomile oil on your sheets and put on soothing music.

6. Turn back your sheets. Appreciate feelings of calm and your anticipation for a good night's sleep.

Helpful Tips:

→ A room divider in the bedroom is a nice way to demark the working and sleeping sections.

→ If your TV is in the bedroom, sit on a chair while watching it. Do not watch television in bed.

Develop a Consistent Sleep Schedule

Waking up at the same time each day is paramount to good sleep. Figure out an optimal wake time by identifying the time you need to begin your workday and working backward. For example, if you need to leave home by 8:00 a.m. and like to have 30 minutes to exercise, 30 minutes to get dressed, and 30 minutes for eating breakfast or other self-care habits, you might wake at 6:30 a.m. This means you would need to go to sleep by 11:30 each night.

1. In month one, focus on waking up at the same time every morning. Set your alarm for the appropriate wake-up time to get your body acclimated.

2. In month two, focus on getting the requisite number of hours of sleep by consistently going to bed at the optimal time. Set an alarm for 30 minutes (or more if needed) before your scheduled bedtime to trigger your awareness that it is time to prepare for bed.

3. In month three, focus on maintaining your sleep schedule. Eventually, you may not need an alarm to remind you to wind down or to wake up.

Notice your increased ability to focus and be creative as a result of getting regular sleep.

Helpful Tips:
→ If you do not fall asleep after 20 minutes or so, get out of bed and do something relaxing until you feel ready to go to sleep. Avoid using your devices and stick with analog pastimes.

→ If you require eight hours of sleep each night, adjust your bedtime to accommodate that need.

Create a Bedtime Ritual

Creating a bedtime ritual that includes relaxing activities is an important self-care habit. When you engage in consistent behaviors before bed, your brain will associate them with sleep, and the signals to wind down and prepare for sleep will become automatic. This habit works in tandem with developing a consistent sleep schedule.

Pick a relaxing activity that you would like to do every night just before bed. This can include listening to soothing music, meditating, writing in your journal, or reading a book. For a week, take an inventory of what you typically do before bed and write it down. Make sure to include weekends. Once you have made your list, notice what helps you relax and what keeps you hyped up. If you do not have any bedtime activities, use the list above.

1. About 30 minutes before bed, take up your activity.
2. If you choose an activity that is not time limited, like reading, take special care to stop at your bedtime.

Appreciate how good you feel having time to wind down, and notice the ease with which you fall asleep when you go to bed already in a relaxed state.

Helpful Tips:
→ It's important that if you choose to read before bed, you read on paper rather than on a screen.

→ If you use your phone as an alarm, do not use it after turning off the alarm.

Take Brief Naps When Needed

Napping can be a tricky thing: most people benefit from taking an afternoon nap, but others find it disruptive to their overall sleep hygiene. Naps can help energize your brain, make you more creative, help you feel refreshed, and even positively impact your immune system. But not all naps can help you. Napping to make up for lost sleep can leave you stuck in a negative cycle, whereas longer naps can throw you off your sleep schedule by inviting the body to go into deep stages of sleep and fragmenting the body's natural sleep rhythms, making it difficult to sleep through the night.

According to the Sleep Foundation, short power naps of 10 to 30 minutes are the most beneficial. If you are someone who is predisposed to taking naps or would like to incorporate naps into your day, keep them short.

1. Set your alarm for 20 minutes and begin your nap.
2. When you wake up, reintegrate yourself back into the world by standing up, stretching, and walking.
3. If you found that 20 minutes was not enough, for your next nap try 25 minutes. Do not exceed 30 minutes at a time.

When you awake, notice how refreshed you feel. Take note of how you perform tasks afterward.

Helpful Tips:

→ Limit your naps to one per day. Frequent naps have a negative impact on your sleep schedule.

→ Don't nap too close to bedtime, and, if possible, do not nap after 3:00 p.m.

Breaking Bad Habits

The first step in breaking bad sleep habits is to surface the negative beliefs that drive the behavior. Take a few moments to write down the beliefs you have about sleep. Notice whether those beliefs are accurate. Are you considering sleep as you need it in your life now? Have you been harboring a belief that operating on a few hours of sleep is a badge of honor? You will likely notice that bad habits are due to outmoded beliefs or patterns that formed in childhood or, more likely, in young adulthood.

I find that many bad habits related to sleep have to do with seeking control when we feel we do not have it—a little rebellion. For example, do you stay up late mindlessly watching television because you want to feel like you have a chance to reclaim the time that you gave to work tasks or family or caretaking responsibilities?

Now that you have clarity about your beliefs, it is time to address your conscious or unconscious rebellion by eliminating some bad sleep habits, like staying on screens too close to bedtime, exercising too close to bedtime, and catching up on sleep on your days off.

Staying on Screens Too Close to Bedtime

You are likely aware of the addictive nature of Internet and smartphone use, but you may be less aware of the negative effects your devices have on your sleep. Electronics emit blue light, which has an excitatory effect on your brain. Blue light blocks the production of melatonin (the sleep hormone), which is typically secreted a couple of hours before bedtime and is a crucial component in getting a good night's sleep. When you're unable to fully enter into deep sleep, the physiological processes that occur during sleep–cell regeneration, healing, and information processing–are not optimally completed. For this reason, it is helpful to break the habit of using screens during the two hours before bed.

1. In week one, stop using your devices (computer, tablet, smartphone, television) 30 minutes before bed.
2. When you feel the urge to use one, tell yourself, "Don't do it," and comply with this self-command.
3. Continue shaving off 30 minutes a week for the next three weeks until you have gotten to two hours.

Helpful Tips:

→ If possible, remove your television and computer from your bedroom and put your phone in a drawer, away from your bed, at night.

→ If you find it too challenging to stop using your phone before bed, dim the brightness setting.

Exercising Too Close to Bedtime

Regular exercise is one of the most effective ways to improve sleep and reduce stress. However, many people don't recognize that failing to pay attention to the timing of your exercise session can bring about sleep problems. In general, it is helpful to finish exercising at least two hours before bedtime.

Exercise makes you more alert and increases the flow of hormones like epinephrine and adrenaline. If you are not aware of the excitatory effect of exercise, you might misattribute your difficulty falling or staying asleep to other factors.

Often, exercising at night is related to how you have managed your time during the day. Incremental changes are an effective way to break this habit.

1. Note the time when you typically exercise and compare it to your typical bedtime.

2. If there is anything less than two hours between the two times, schedule your workout to start 15 minutes earlier the following week. When you're done, congratulate yourself!

3. The next time you exercise, start 15 minutes earlier than you did the last time and continue to move up your evening exercise in 15-minute increments until there is at least two hours between when you finish exercising and when you go to bed.

Helpful Tips:
→ Some people can sleep just after exercising, so it is important to know what works for you.

→ If you take hot baths at night after working out, you'll need to make sure that your exercise and your bath are completed two hours before bed, since such baths energize you rather than provide calm.

Trying to Catch Up on Sleep on Your Days Off

"I'm so tired, I can't wait until the weekend when I can catch up on sleep!" How many times have you said some version of that? One reason that people are so cavalier about lack of sleep during the week is because they plan to compensate for their poor sleep habits on their days off. This behavior provides a false sense of recovery. That temporary relief actually results in a hard-to-repay sleep debt and continues a vicious cycle. For example, sleeping in on Saturday and then staying up late that night because you're not sleepy at your regular bedtime pushes your whole sleep schedule back. When you sleep in again on Sunday, you will also not be sleepy at bedtime on Sunday night—but you will still have to get up Monday morning. Consequently, you'll feel tired from lack of sleep. Then you'll spend the week trying to regain lost sleep and normalize your sleep schedule, only to throw it all out of whack again when the weekend comes.

1. Decide whether you will wake up at your regular time on Saturday or allow yourself up to one hour of extra sleep on the weekend. Set your alarm for the time you decided on.
2. Wake up when the alarm goes off and get up. Do not press snooze.

3. Relish the fact that you are engaging in sleep hygiene.

4. Take one 20-minute nap the next afternoon and as needed over the next few days to stay energized.

Helpful Tip:

→ If you want to recover from lost sleep, add in extra sleep in small increments over the course of a few days to get back on track.

Tracking Your Progress

Use this tracker as a tool to help you monitor your progress and gain insight into why a habit perhaps isn't quite sticking. We track our habits so we can learn, modify, and improve.

HABIT	M	T	W	TH	F	SAT	S

KEY TAKEAWAYS

- Building good sleep hygiene is the quickest and most effective way to shift your current feelings of well-being.

- You likely formed your approach to sleep as a child or adolescent. Therefore, you may have some ill-informed thoughts and behaviors around sleep. It's time to think of sleep as something that supports your adult self.

- Sleeping well has a great deal to do with what you do before going to bed. Once you shift your mindset to incorporate this awareness, you'll be better equipped to make positive changes to your sleep habits.

- Stack the habits listed in this chapter to develop strong sleep hygiene.

CHAPTER 7

Taking a Break

It is commonly accepted that relaxing is an important aspect of life. Yet moments of relaxation are often seen as special occasion activities that require getting away from our everyday lives. For many, weekends are the key to becoming rejuvenated, but let's face it: weekends are often full of errands, games, and household chores. All of these are necessary activities, so I invite you to counterbalance them with daily and weekly activities that will allow you to feel more rested and rejuvenated to further strengthen your self-care. In this chapter, I will share simple strategies such as taking daily breaks to improve your life.

Why Taking Breaks and Relaxation Matter

At a purely physical level, the body requires periods of recovery. Drs. Emily and Amelia Nagoski, in their ground-breaking book *Burnout: The Secret to Unlocking the Stress Cycle,* call these recovery periods "rest." They believe that resting is really body renewal, the formula for unlocking the stress cycle. Further, their research suggests that the body needs 42 percent of a 24-hour day (roughly 10 hours including sleep) to be spent at rest; without it, over time, there will be serious physical and emotional repercussions.

This book is about cultivating habits that balance several important spheres of life. Taking breaks and creating moments of rest and relaxation is the very essence of the guiding definition of self-care. In that sense, rest for rest's sake has a positive impact on general well-being, mood, physical health, productivity, creativity, and the ability to meet life's challenges.

Internal medicine physician Dr. Saundra Dalton-Smith describes the need for seven types of rest: physical, creative, spiritual, emotional, sensory, social, and mental. Suffice it to say, every part of you needs to be nurtured and restored by moments of rest. Figuring out what type of rest you need and then tailoring your schedule to meet that need is imperative. In this chapter, I will recommend various types of rest for your consideration. I encourage you to think of relaxation and rest in doses, almost like vitamins or medication. You can have microdoses, such as short breaks during the day, or a macrodose that includes a weeklong vacation. What's important is that you recognize that breaks are as necessary as your daily hygiene activities.

Building Healthier Habits

You might associate relaxation with popular self-care activities like spa visits, meditation, or yoga retreats. Although such activities that provide respite from everyday life are useful strategies, they aren't the only strategies. There are many easy daily habits that can help you build rest and relaxation into your life.

I have often recommended that the college students I work with take scheduled breaks while studying, because it helps enhance their attention and reduce stress. And less stress overall helps academic performance. Taking a dedicated relaxation break during the day, whether it be from caregiving, office work, or schoolwork, can have a positive effect on how you approach your labor and reduce stress overall. Although the goal of breaks and relaxation is not solely to increase performance, it is helpful to recognize the link between the two in order to counteract any beliefs you might hold that taking a break would negatively impact your performance. You can be a "good" parent and take a break. You can be a dedicated club volunteer and set boundaries on the time you give. Thinking that things will fall apart if you take a break is a trap many people fall into, especially when they experience the rush of adrenaline that can come when pushing through stress signals in the name of reaching goals.

The habits in this chapter will help you build rest into your life, help you learn to say no, and help you give yourself permission to take breaks.

Say No

In Western society, it can seem like everyone—including family, professional contacts, and social acquaintances—consciously or unconsciously subscribes to the notion that a dedication to work and productivity is paramount. In some cases, this can result in overcommitment and even burnout. At its core, it also opens the door to a belief that your worth is tied to others' approval.

Active self-compassion is a powerful antidote to this thinking, because it allows you to let your self-concept remain constant and not fall prey to others' judgment. Setting boundaries and saying no to requests for your time is one of the most self-compassionate things you can do for your well-being.

1. Schedule and block out an hour each day to do something that is relaxing.
2. When something comes up or you get an invitation that overlaps with your relaxation time, say no. Protect this time.
3. Continue this weekly for two months.
4. Take stock of how this boundary setting opens up time for other self-care.
5. Once this habit has been ingrained, work to only place things on your calendar that don't interfere with your personal time.

Enjoy the rest and relaxation that you allow yourself. Notice how it affects your energy level, performance, and stress level. Embrace the sense of empowerment you've gained from protecting your personal time.

→ Tell your friends and family that you are practicing self-care by streamlining your schedule, and you would like their help in taking on a task and will begin to delegate some responsibilities.

Take Breaks During the Day

I encourage you to think of regular breaks throughout your day not as an indulgence but rather as a regular practice that feels good and is good for you. In *Success: The Psychology of Achievement*, Deborah Olson highlights a study by the Draugium Group that found the most productive employees took a 17-minute break about every 52 minutes of work per day. Those who took breaks were more motivated to do their work and better able to prioritize tasks. This advice reinforces the notion that just "powering through" the day or a challenging project or assignment likely does not yield the most effective outcomes.

Scheduling in advance during your day can be helpful and can lessen the likelihood that you work to a place of exhaustion. Let's begin a daily habit toward work breaks during the morning.

1. Schedule a recurring 15-minute break in your calendar during each work or school day.

2. Move away from your workstation or desk to give yourself a change of scenery.

3. Determine if you will take a walk or engage in a relaxation exercise. Do not check emails or spend the time texting.

4. After two months, move to two morning breaks a day.

Notice how much better you are able to focus after your break.

Helpful Tips:

→ If you are retired or do not currently work, breaks are still meaningful and important. Plan a break during your day using the above strategy.

→ If you have shift work and are not in control of when you can take a break, use the same principles for how to spend your time when you are scheduled for a break.

Take a Tech Break

Blue light and bright light are helpful in compelling alertness; however, as you might imagine, constant use of electronics and tech tools keeps your mind active even when you're attempting periods of rest. It might be that you need a complete break from your computer or phone, especially if you spend most of your day working on one.

For this example, please consider refraining from using your computer, smartphone, tablet, television, or gaming system.

1. Set aside one hour each weekend (or any day you typically try to rest) to go tech-free. Let your loved ones and friends know in advance.
2. Pick an alternate tech-free activity to do with others or by yourself (crossword puzzle, card or board game, reading a book, etc.).
3. When you have the urge to turn on or reach for the item, tell yourself, "Don't do it."
4. Celebrate your success!

Although this may feel difficult at first, pay attention to how your tech-free activity increases your attention span and focus over time. You may also find that you learned something new or increased your skill in that activity.

Helpful Tips:
→ If possible, put away the tech item during your break or move to another room so you are not tempted.

→ If you are a heavy tech user, roll this back to smaller steps, starting with 30 seconds without picking up your phone and working up to an hour.

Meditate

Meditation has a variety of benefits in addition to providing rest–think reduced stress, improved attention span, decreased blood pressure, and improved mood.

If you have tried meditation before but stopped after a few attempts, thinking you were not good at it or were unable to quiet your mind, I encourage you to try again with a different type of meditation that may be better for you. This is the type of endeavor that is about practice, not perfection.

Begin by scheduling meditation at the same time every day—I recommend first thing in the morning right before breakfast. To start, meditate in the same place, such as your favorite chair.

1. During the first week, at the appointed time, go to the place you selected and set a timer for two minutes. Close your eyes and breathe in and out at your own pace. As you inhale, silently say to yourself, "I am breathing in," and on the exhale say, "I am breathing out."
2. During week two, continue this practice, but extend the time to five minutes.
3. During week three, add two minutes to complete seven minutes.
4. During week four, progress to a ten-minute session.

Notice and appreciate increased feelings of centeredness and improved mood.

Helpful Tips:

→ Choose a calming chime as the timer ringer on your phone for this exercise.

→ The goal is not to quiet your mind but to focus on your breathing. If you get distracted, simply go back to your breath.

→ If this still feels too challenging after you have tried for a bit, search for a guided meditation app.

Breaking Bad Habits

Tara, a high-powered tech executive, was used to working around the clock brokering international deals. When I recommended that she take breaks during the day, her feelings of discomfort and distress were palpable. Imagine that a roller coaster car stopped suddenly, the brakes having been hit mid-ride. The force of the stop would be jarring to the occupants not only because they didn't expect it but also because their body would continue moving. A break can feel this alarming for those who are overwhelmed and habituated to nonstop demands on their time. In the beginning, breaks may provoke a feeling of discomfort. Many people, regardless of what their job is or what demands are made of them in modern life, feel much like Tara on the roller coaster.

Difficulty taking a break is often due to knowing yourself best based on who you are to others and what you do for others. Rest is time with yourself, and if you aren't accustomed to that time, it can sometimes feel like a blind date. This feeling can change, and addressing the following habits can help you on that journey.

Not Separating Work and Home Life

It's easy to carry your work and other responsibilities around with you, thinking about them even when you're not engaged in your tasks. In this case, you need a mindset shift: you can be more relaxed and engaged in your daily life if you take a real break off-hours. I find that I can easily make this shift during planned vacations, so I imagine the end of my workday as stepping into a mini vacation.

Doing so gives me permission to transition to my personal time. Here, let's focus on doing a brain dump after work.

1. Choose a comfortable place in your home. Each day, at a consistent time, soon after your daily responsibilities end, make this the first place you go.

2. Take a few moments to dump all of your thoughts into a notebook or the notes app on your phone. No need to edit, as the list can consist of to-do items for the next day, frustrations, and inspirations. Take a few moments to write it all out.

3. After that, when you start to think about school or work or have an urge to check your email, tell yourself, "Don't do it," and take three deep cleansing breaths.

Helpful Tip:
→ If you struggle with checking work email, try unsaving your password. Having to enter the password manually requires you to pause for a beat and can be a helpful deterrent.

Working through Lunch

Life was likely easier when the bell rang to signal it was your lunch period and you spent that time eating and playing. As adults, many people either continue working while they eat or don't eat at all.

I'm here to tell you that lunch breaks are necessary at all stages of life. They provide time for rejuvenation and improve work satisfaction. Here is a plan for how you can begin to break the habit of working through lunch using the power of accountability.

1. Find an accountability buddy (or two) to have lunch with during the work week. Ask if they would be willing to commit to having lunch away from their desks for two months.

2. Agree on a shared lunch break time and add it to your calendar. Set a reminder to go off 15 minutes before your break to remind you it is time to begin winding down the work you are doing.

3. Recognize how energized you are for the rest of the day.

4. Be diligent about not scheduling meetings during this time.

Helpful Tips:

→ If you work in shifts, get several lunch buddies.

→ If you have a 30-minute break, it is helpful to bring your lunch rather than spend time purchasing. Consider other time management measures as needed.

→ If you work from home or by yourself, ask someone in your life to call you at lunch to support you in stepping away for your break. Alternatively, you can text them to confirm that you are taking lunch.

Failure to Give Yourself Respite

In an ideal world, we would all get a vacation from our paid and unpaid labor, including caregiving, but that is not the case for a significant portion of the population. For many people, including college students, people who string together part-time jobs to make ends meet, family caregivers, entrepreneurs, and office workers, there are a multitude of reasons why an extended period of rest seems impossible. Reasons include lack of other family members to share caretaking duties with, discouragement from bosses, or cultural messages that we ought to be productive at all times.

As you think of your self-respite, especially if you do not often do so, it is helpful to create time to simply be rather than to do or produce. Allot a three-hour chunk of time per month to do "nothing." If you are a caretaker, ask a trusted friend or other family member to give you a respite break. You can trade off and offer the same to that person when they take a respite break.

1. Plan in advance how you will spend your time, including lots of downtime. Do not overbook yourself. You can schedule a pampering appointment, sit in a café and people watch, or go to a park and enjoy your surroundings.

2. At the appointed time, take your break.

3. Notice your discomfort, if any, and say, "It's okay; I deserve time to myself."

4. Repeat this practice and build up to two respite days per month, if you are able.

Helpful Tip:
→ Consider what plans you might need to put in place to make this happen.

Tracking Your Progress

Use this tracker as a tool to help you monitor your progress and gain insight into why a habit perhaps isn't quite sticking. We track our habits so we can learn, modify, and improve.

HABIT	M	T	W	TH	F	SAT	S

KEY TAKEAWAYS

- Breaks and relaxation do not need to be relegated to special occasions; you can find daily ways to give yourself rest. Aim for 10 hours of rest each day (including sleep).

- You require different forms of rest. Use the variety of suggestions in this chapter to bolster yourself in the ways you most need.

- There can be personal, familial, and professional expectations that keep you from giving yourself opportunities to relax. Find people in your life who support your becoming more relaxed and want to do the same.

- You might find relaxing or taking breaks uncomfortable at first. This discomfort can be emotional or physical. It doesn't mean anything is wrong—you are simply building a new habit. Start slowly and work to add more as your comfort level rises.

- Try to schedule at least one longer break per month to allow yourself to recharge.

CHAPTER 8

Practicing Self-Compassion

Your relationship with yourself is at the foundation of every other relationship in your life. It's commonly said that when you love yourself, you demonstrate to others how you expect to be treated. This truism is important, yet it is not the full story. Loving yourself requires accepting the totality of who you are, what makes you fabulous and what makes you flawed. Self-compassion is an important element of self-care, because without it, you can easily fall prey to self-judgment that stalls your willingness to take care of yourself. In this chapter, I'll discuss how to develop self-compassion habits to help cultivate self-care.

Why Self-Compassion Matters

Throughout the book, I have encouraged you to bring a nonjudgmental stance to evaluating your current level of self-care. In lieu of judgment, I have asked you to be curious. Self-compassion is a key ingredient to supporting a nonjudgmental stance, because it allows you to look at yourself, see the totality of your experience, and accept yourself. Doing this requires the same compassion you would give to a loved one, a beloved child, or a best friend.

Self-compassion is a concept often discussed in Buddhist teachings and practices. It was popularized nearly 20 years ago in psychology by Dr. Kristin Neff, who researched self-compassion and its components, which include self-kindness, common humanity, and mindfulness. In a nutshell, these components lead you to release self-criticism, understand that your imperfection unifies you with others (makes you no different from others), and allows you to face your pain rather than believe it is indicative of your worth.

If you want to improve your relationship with yourself and with others, start with self-compassion. For, as you can imagine, it is challenging to give others what you cannot give yourself. Benefits of self-compassion include a lower likelihood of depression and anxiety, as well as increased positivity. Noted researcher and author Dr. Brené Brown has linked self-compassion to personal bravery. As you might imagine, the self-acceptance that accompanies self-compassion leads to greater life satisfaction and overall well-being. This practice can help you face obstacles and recover from challenges with more equanimity.

Building Healthier Habits

At the heart of self-compassion is increasing your self-awareness through noticing your experience. You might find that the benefit of these observations is a deepened relationship with yourself. As you begin to understand your unique emotional landscape, you might notice feeling lighter and more liberated. To be honest, you might also find it a bit scary, because you may find out some things about yourself that you might not like. Often, I find that people can live in extremes—deeply immersed in their emotional experience or totally tuned out. Some may have grown up in circumstances where they were told they were not good enough, informing their self-perception in the present. I want to make sure to acknowledge that impaired self-perception can relate to previous trauma, health issues, and mental health concerns. In such cases, it is most appropriate to seek the help of a trained professional to guide you through the process of self-discovery and also help you offset the potential emotional impact of uncovering deeply stored pain.

The habits in this chapter are meant to deepen your self-compassion by drawing awareness to the totality of your experience.

Write in a Journal

The act of journaling—writing out your thoughts, feelings, and experiences—can help you detach from events that have happened and create a bit of distance from them in order to cultivate your self-compassion. For this habit, you will practice perspective-taking by writing about your day using the prompts below. You will practice giving yourself the same compassion you might give a friend.

1. Designate a consistent time to reflect on the day.
2. Record a significant feeling you had. Try using a sentence like, *Today I felt [emotion] because of [event].* Repeat this habit every day at the same time for one week.
3. At the end of one week, read through your notes and assess your reflections for negative self-appraisal or judgment.
4. If you feel dismayed or upset by what you have recorded, imagine how you might feel if someone you care for wrote about themselves in such a way. Record how you would support them.

When you reread your notes, notice that you can look upon your experiences with an increased sense of peace.

Helpful Tips:

→ You can add this practice to your pre-bedtime ritual. I have found that it can help my clients sleep more easily when they release stressors onto the page.

→ If you do not already have a journaling practice and feel like you do not have much to say, write for five minutes and build up over time.

Repeat Positive Affirmations

Focusing on what you want in your life rather than what you do not want is a powerful way to create change. The truth is, negative thoughts about yourself, or focusing on what is wrong, can lead to an imbalanced perspective of yourself. I invite you to use affirmations as you begin to reprogram your thoughts toward self-compassion.

Affirmations are short, positive phrases said repeatedly to shift your thinking to a new state. They can be done any time of day, yet doing them in the morning can have a powerful effect. Start by writing a few affirmations like these on sticky notes and putting them where you will see them often: *I accept myself as I am, I am kind to myself, I allow myself to grow and learn each day,* and *It's okay to make mistakes and learn from them.*

1. Pair reading your affirmations aloud with a daily task you spend a few minutes doing. For example, if the task is grooming, place the affirmation on your bathroom mirror. If it is dressing, place them on your bedroom mirror.
2. Read three of your affirmations aloud.
3. Notice how you feel after reading each affirmation.
4. Congratulate yourself each day for doing this activity.

As you savor the positive emotions that come from reading the affirmations, you may also feel more optimistic.

Helpful Tips:
→ If you find it challenging to say the affirmation because it is too far from what you currently

believe, add the phrase "I am in the process of . . ."
For instance, "I am in the process of accepting
myself as I am."

→ Add new affirmations over time.

Give Yourself a Hug

For this habit, you will practice self-soothing in challenging moments. I often recommend this strategy to my clients when they are judging themselves for their reactions. It can be deeply useful to know that you can give yourself what you crave. If you grew up in an environment where adults did not know how to soothe your big emotions or teach you how to do so, then this habit is for you.

Think about a time when you were feeling upset. Not greatly upset, but enough to know you felt different from your baseline. Allow yourself to bring up thoughts and emotions from that time. Now give yourself a hug by placing your right hand on your left arm and your left hand on your right arm. Give your upper arms a gentle squeeze, then stroke your upper arms by guiding them from your elbows to upper shoulders. You just gave yourself a hug!

1. The next time you experience challenging or painful emotions or have negative thoughts about yourself, pause and notice.
2. Give yourself a hug.
3. Pair the hug with the statement, "This is a moment of suffering, and it's okay."

After the statement, you may gain a sense of calm and your body may feel at peace.

→ Pair this activity with journaling.

→ You can adjust this habit and do it daily rather than in a moment of suffering.

Practice Gratitude

In some ways, gratitude is about looking at either the silver lining or the lessons from a situation. It is an effective way to create change in your perception of your life. Gratitude can allow you to take a fuller look at all aspects of your life. The goal is not to pretend suffering does not exist but to recognize that it can coexist with joy.

For this practice you are going to use a common positive psychology exercise called "Three Good Things." To do it, you will practice identifying three good things that happened during your day. You will use a few prompts to further explore each of those three things.

1. Pick an already ingrained habit that you do each night to stack with this habit. For example, after cleaning up from dinner or just before your bedtime ritual.

2. Write down your three good things.

3. Use these prompts to analyze each good thing:
   What went well today was _____.
   It went well because _____.

4. Read your responses aloud and let them sink in.

As you take stock of how much there is to be grateful for right now, you may feel an increased appreciation for life and a sense of calm and perspective.

Helpful Tips:

→ If this doesn't come naturally, don't worry; over time it will become easier.

→ Consider sharing your list with a friend.

Breaking Bad Habits

Limited self-compassion can have many origins. You may have grown up in challenging circumstances where you were not afforded the benefit of being told positive things about yourself. You may have been in competitive or high-achievement environments or spent years in school where you were constantly given feedback about how you needed to be better. Such environments can tear away at a person's self-image and lead to a false belief that self-compassion takes away the competitive edge.

Researchers Dr. Nicola Hermanto and Dr. David Charles Zuroff explored the relationship between self-compassion and caregiving, which is worth noting. In a 2016 study of 195 college students, they found that those who reported the least self-compassion also engaged in the highest level of caregiving. This matches my clinical experience, in that many of the people I have worked with who dedicate their lives to taking care of others have been woefully bad at taking care of themselves. This tendency has been termed "compulsive caregiving"– giving to others while simultaneously having difficulty allowing themselves to receive from others. The habits you will focus on breaking in this chapter are failing to counterbalance negative judgments, trying to be perfect, and comparing yourself to others. These are all common habits that have a way of sneaking into your life and eroding your self-image, and each can be changed through awareness, vigilant monitoring, and, most important, self-compassion.

Failure to Counterbalance Negative Judgment

When something challenging or hurtful occurs in adult life, you may find yourself responding in a way that you find surprising—and then judge yourself, often through negative self-statements. A negative self-statement is an automatic, negative appraisal of yourself, such as "I'm so clumsy."

Much of your response in these circumstances stems from your emotional history. Psychologists agree that a person's typical constellation of emotional reactions is formed in childhood. Thus, it should not be a shock that times of stress can activate an emotional response from that time, even in a 25-, 45-, or 65-year-old person. Do not judge yourself when you have those reactions. First notice your reaction. Then give yourself grace and allow for the possibility that you can create a new pattern.

1. In week one, notice your reactions during stressful situations and write down your negative self-statements.

2. In week two, continue to write down any negative self-statements that arise, but now, counterbalance each one with a self-compassionate statement, such as *I trip sometimes and that is okay* or *I allow myself to be perfectly imperfect.*

→ If it's hard to write a self-compassionate statement, imagine making the compassionate statement to a loved one.

→ If you cannot give compassion to your adult self, give compassion to your child self.

Trying to Be Perfect

Perfection is simply not possible. Even if you do not consciously think of yourself as trying to be perfect, it can show up in the energy you put into avoiding mistakes. Guess what—mistakes are a natural part of life. Recognizing this fact can provide a sense of freedom.

When you aim for perfection, you block your innate ability to grow and learn as fully as you might otherwise. Learning is often developed through failure and stretching yourself beyond what is comfortable. To break the habit of perfectionism, try something new that you know will lead to mistakes, then purposefully observe, learn from, and give yourself grace when you make them.

Pick something in your life you have always wanted to learn that does not come naturally for you. For example, drawing, painting, or sewing.

1. Schedule a time for the activity you picked.

2. Give yourself permission to do it imperfectly.

3. Notice how you feel when you make a mistake. Compare how you thought it would be versus how it turned out.

4. Ask yourself what you can learn from the mistake.

5. Move on from the mistake and return to the activity.

Helpful Tips:

→ If you feel so inclined, share your final product with someone and ask for feedback.

→ If you continue practicing this activity, over time you will improve. Notice that you are still the same person as you were when you started; what has changed is your perspective.

Drawing Unfair Comparisons

I am sure this will not come as a surprise, but social media does not offer an accurate perspective of the lives of others. Even so-called "no filter" posts are carefully curated. And that is totally fine. The problem comes when, despite knowing this, you compare your life to what you see online. This is a reality of the social media age, and the strategy is not to totally avoid it (unless of course that feels good to you) but rather to put it in its proper place. In order to do so, in this habit, you will send yourself compassion.

1. While on social media, notice when you start to compare yourself negatively to others, feel envy, or have general unease.

2. When this happens, take the opportunity to silently send positive thoughts to the other person and to yourself. You might say, "I honor you and I honor me. I wish you peace, and I wish myself peace."

3. Repeat this each time the feelings arise.

Helpful Tip:

→ If you find yourself envious of facets of other people's lives, it might signal your desire to make changes in your own life. If this is the case, redirect your energy toward putting a plan in place for how you will accomplish your goals.

Tracking Your Progress

Use this tracker as a tool to help you monitor your progress and gain insight into why a habit perhaps isn't quite sticking. We track our habits so we can learn, modify, and improve.

HABIT	M	T	W	TH	F	SAT	S

KEY TAKEAWAYS

- Self-compassion allows you to remember that you deserve the same care you offer loved ones.

- A key to self-compassion is increasing your self-awareness, which allows you to become more deeply acquainted with your full emotional landscape. Labeling your emotions and writing in a journal are strong tactics for better understanding.

- Undoubtedly, you will have emotions and experiences that feel challenging. You can self-soothe by giving yourself a hug, practicing gratitude, and using affirmations.

- Perfection is an illusion. Media—including social media—provides an airbrushed version of life. If you don't counterbalance or take a break from these images, the cycle of perfectionism and self-judgment will continue.

- Self-compassion requires ongoing attention and lifelong practice, so keep at it!

CHAPTER 9

Managing Stress

S tress is a normal part of daily life. It's what helps you to get up each day and care enough to participate in daily activities. Stress and the energy it offers are fuel for achieving personal and professional goals. But stress sustained at moderate to high levels is not meant to be a common factor of life, and leads to burnout. In this chapter, I'll focus on self-care as a strategy to recover from sustained stress and to mitigate the possibility of burnout.

Why Managing Stress Matters

Note the key idea here is *managing* stress. Stress isn't a bad thing in and of itself; it is your body's normal reaction to daily life, helping to marshal your reactions to accomplish all the tasks it needs to do to help you live happily and healthily. In normal life, most stressors you face are mild to moderate ones. They're just enough to activate the sympathetic nervous system and get you up and doing whatever it is you need to do. When you're finished dealing with the stressor, the parasympathetic nervous system takes over and allows you to recover. When this happens and you complete the stress cycle, you are managing stress successfully.

The problem happens when you are under constant or severe stress. In this situation, it's common to adopt some habits that are supposed to help you cope, but that never actually manage to resolve the stress. When stress is not addressed and the cycle remains unresolved, it puts your body under long-term strain, overloading your defense mechanisms, making you susceptible to disease, and basically causing the body to break down.

In this chapter, I'll help you get off the stress roller coaster by explaining how you can manage your stress with the help of healthy habits. You'll also learn to identify common bad habits and learn strategies for breaking them.

Building Healthier Habits

There is an inverse relationship that stress can have with performance. Each person has their own specific performance level where they perform optimally, but each person also has their own level at which stress becomes too great and performance starts to go down.

Since a life without any stress at all is an impossibility (and one you actually do not want), what you want to do is recognize, appreciate, and respond appropriately to your own stress levels. As this chapter progresses, you'll be exposed to a variety of habits that are among my go-to strategies for helping my clients develop their own plan for how they respond to stress. You will learn how to use at least one of the following habits to complete your stress cycle. You will also learn to set boundaries so you can remain at your optimal performance level.

Take Breathing Breaks

One of the first self-care practices I encourage my clients to start with is deep breathing. Deep belly breathing has been shown to be an effective stress management measure in moments of mild to moderate distress. Without realizing it, most people (without breathing issues) breathe shallowly and therefore have not experienced the benefits of deep belly breathing.

For this habit, you will create breathing breaks over the course of your day and pair them with a regular task, such as leaving the restroom or walking to get the mail. In this practice, you will take three deep breaths.

1. After exiting the bathroom or on your way to the mail, pause where you are and take a deep breath. Breathe in through your nose and let your belly fill with air, then move your breath up your chest, filling your lungs to a count of five.
2. Pause at the top of the breath for one to two counts.
3. Exhale slowly through your mouth for a count of eight (or until you have released all the air in your belly).
4. Repeat this two more times.

As you continue on your way, notice the feeling of warmth and relaxation you have gained.

Helpful Tips:

→ You'll find that, over time, you'll start to do this naturally.

→ Feel free to pair your breaths with a different activity.

→ There are a variety of breathing activities and practices you can do. Feel free to substitute one that you like better and follow the implementation plan I've described.

Label Your Emotions

Stress is a general term often associated with a series of emotions, such as frustration, overwhelm, worry, and irritation. It is helpful to note that your feelings are not singular—often they are a constellation of emotions that exist concurrently. For this habit, you will label your emotions when you are feeling chronic or situational stress that is unresolved.

1. When you encounter a stressful situation that requires problem-solving, pause for a few moments and write down the emotions you're feeling in your journal or in the notes section of your phone.
2. Think about what makes the situation stressful.
3. Then take a few moments to brainstorm possible solutions to the problem. Look for solutions to the stressor.
4. Pick a solution, or a combination of solutions, from your list and proceed toward resolving your stress.
5. Congratulate yourself for tending to your emotions.

You likely gained a release from some of the stress that you're feeling just by labeling the emotions. Enjoy the space that release allows you to problem solve.

Helpful Tip:
→ Doing this exercise "as is" will prove to be useful. If you would like to take it a step further, look at your list of emotions and see if you might focus on the lighter or neutral emotions. Sometimes that is a helpful strategy to recognize that every situation is more than one thing or has more than one aspect.

Attend to Your Body

Because emotional aspects of stress, such as feeling overwhelmed, burned out, or unmotivated, are often felt so deeply, people often end up tuning out altogether. In doing so, they often tune out to the care their body needs after navigating daily life. As such, it is useful to develop a habit of giving your body daily TLC at the end of each day to help resolve any leftover vestiges of stress.

In *Burnout: The Secret to Unlocking the Stress Cycle,* Drs. Emily and Amelia Nagoski describe physical activity as "the single most efficient strategy for completing the stress cycle." They further identify that traditional forms of exercise are not the only way to mitigate stress. You can also do so by tensing and relaxing your muscles as you breathe. This strategy, called progressive relaxation, is a popular technique that mental health practitioners frequently teach clients. You will develop this habit by paying attention to your physical symptoms of stress. You can also draw from the many habits listed in chapter 3 for additional inspiration if you prefer other forms of exercise.

1. At the conclusion of your daily tasks, have a seat or lie down.
2. Starting with your shoulders and moving down until you arrive at your feet, inhale while tensing your muscle groups, one at a time, and exhale as you release your muscles.
3. Congratulate yourself for taking this important step toward resolving your stress!

Savor how much lighter and more relaxed your body feels after giving it this additional TLC.

Helpful Tip:
→ If your daytime schedule is quite stressful, consider this exercise in the afternoon.

Laugh

Have you have ever felt down or been in a bad mood, but then someone unexpectedly told a joke, or you read something funny, and found yourself busting out in laughter? If so, your mood likely improved from that moment of levity. Not only does laughter improve mood, but it has also been found to reduce pain, support immunity, and benefit heart health. So let's not leave moments of laughter up to chance.

A 2015 study in *Evidence-Based Complementary and Alternative Medicine* yielded some interesting results regarding the link between laughter and stress symptoms among people receiving treatment for cancer. Participants joined four sessions of a laughter intervention, and after a single session, it effectively reduced anxiety, depression, and stress.

Start by listing what you know makes you laugh, and be open to exploring other things that may make you laugh. For example, do you like lighthearted sitcoms, comedy specials, adorable cat videos, satire, or humorous books? Pick one item from your list to try.

1. At a time of day when you generally need a boost to your mood, watch or read the thing you chose from your list.
2. Give yourself 30 minutes to enjoy the laughter and release that is produced by the thing on your list.
3. Repeat this five days a week for a month.

Revel in the joy and release that you've gained from loosening the grip of stress with laughter.

→ This is an uplifting habit to incorporate into the time you spend with your significant other, if it is something you can watch or listen to together.

→ A common stressor is watching or reading the news. Balance your news consumption with this laughter habit.

Breaking Bad Habits

As situations that lend themselves to unresolved stress are an ever-present part of Western life, it is shockingly simple to develop bad habits related to stress. It's easy to adopt a belief that since stress is a part of life, there is nothing you can do except push through it.

Many bad habits related to stress are actually behaviors people engage in to mask their stress signals. The most common habits I see are handling stress on one's own and becoming addicted to the rush of last-minute work.

This can show up in the form of numbing behaviors, such as eating when you're not hungry, drinking alcohol, recreational drug use, binge-watching television, Internet use, and gaming. All of these behaviors have the potential to become addictive and can signal a deeper problem that warrants professional support.

Behavioral rehearsal is a change strategy you will be utilizing in this section that allows you to practice a new desired way of being without the stress of the context where it will later be practiced. This is beneficial because it allows you to plan for how to deal with emotional or physical obstacles.

Ignoring Your Stress Signals

I regularly ask my stress management workshop participants to list their stress signals. Most people are intimately acquainted with the indicators that they are stressed, including tightness in their shoulders, gastrointestinal distress, or grumpiness; yet they are less practiced at noticing and then *responding* to those signals. Instead, many people push through their stress signals.

If you notice any of these indicators, then take a moment and write down the things you can do to respond to stressors in the moment. You can draw from the various habit suggestions throughout this book.

1. Create a list of five self-care strategies you can turn to when feeling stress.
2. Think of a situation in the recent past when you felt mild to moderate stress. Recall what you experienced in your body at that time and write it down.
3. Practice one of the self-care strategies from your list with the stressor in mind.
4. Once you are done, notice how you feel. Did your stress increase, decrease, or stay the same?
5. Try each one of the strategies on your list and then rank them. The next time you experience stress in real life, use one of the strategies you practiced.

→ Keep the list in your pocket or handbag or on your phone so it is readily available.

Keeping Your Stress to Yourself

The role personal connection plays in self-care cannot be overstated, as relationships are essential for well-being. There are a variety of reasons that people decide not to let others know they are stressed. For some, there are cultural prohibitions against telling someone outside of your family that you are stressed out. Others may have received messages that falling prey to stress is a sign of personal weakness.

It is helpful to find people you can trust and who give you the type of support you need. For this habit, identify a nurture buddy: someone you can talk to daily and who agrees to share what is going on in their life. If you don't have anyone you can confide in or you need a greater level of support, search for a professional.

1. Pick a time each day to talk. Agree with your nurture buddy that you will take 15 minutes daily to share with each other what happened in the day.
2. Have the conversation. Share as you are comfortable.
3. Notice how giving and receiving support is beneficial to the both of you.

Helpful Tips:
→ The more transparent you are about how you feel, the more benefit you will likely derive from these conversations.

→ To the extent that you can, it is useful to have a few nurture buddies and sources of support that you access on a regular basis.

→ Consider utilizing the services of a therapist, coach, or faith leader. There are supplemental services to connect to in your community.

Not Recognizing You Are Addicted to Stress

Although reducing stress and its impact is a goal many people have, for some, the adrenaline rush that comes from achieving "the impossible" makes it tough for them to do so because they feel they do their best work under pressure. When living with heightened stress becomes a lifestyle, it will eventually catch up with you.

To break this cycle, you must recognize stressful situations exist but do not have to consume your life. Be curious about the impact. This is another opportunity to practice behavioral rehearsal, which has been shown to be very effective at breaking habits like these.

1. Think of a time in your recent past when you felt stressed by all the commitments in your life. What was it about that period that was most challenging? Write down your answers.

2. In your mind's eye, recall being back in that time, but imagine making different decisions that might lower your stress level. Allow yourself to see what comes up and write about it. Feel free to try different options and notice what felt best.

3. Use what you learn from this exercise to plan how you might approach your responsibilities or goal attainment in a more sustainable way. Write it down and mentally rehearse your plan to prepare for next time.

Helpful Tips:

→ This behavioral rehearsal exercise works well when you have an accountability partner.

→ Of course, there are times when you may not be able to escape this type of stress, and that is okay.

Tracking Your Progress

Use this tracker as a tool to help you monitor your progress and gain insight into why a habit perhaps isn't quite sticking. We track our habits so we can learn, modify, and improve.

HABIT	M	T	W	TH	F	SAT	S

KEY TAKEAWAYS

- Stress is a common component of human existence. Your stress response is meant to help you recognize and respond to danger. After acute moments of stress, you are meant to recuperate and restore. This allows you to complete the stress cycle.

- Your brain and body don't differentiate between physical and emotional stressors. In both cases, your sympathetic nervous system springs into action to respond to the threat. So, to your brain, life stressors can feel like you are responding to a physical attack.

- You need your own reliable set of regular self-care habits to face and respond to the stress in your life. Physical activity and talking to someone are among the best habits to develop.

- By becoming aware of your unique stress signals, you can better respond to stress in the moment and lessen its impact.

- Don't let the fact that stress is a normal part of life keep you from addressing it.

CHAPTER 10

Practicing Mindfulness

Mindfulness is an approach to life and behaviors: it is the practice of bringing awareness to the present moment rather than focusing on the past or forecasting the future. Mindfulness is paying attention without judgment about what is happening in the moment. This practice has helped people gain greater insight into themselves and deepen their intuition.

Here, you will focus on how to direct your attention to being more engaged with the present moment. We will also discuss how to minimize the bad habits of living in the past and the future while being oblivious to what's happening right now.

Why Practicing Mindfulness Matters

Think about how you spent the last 24 hours. How much time was spent multitasking, worrying about what might happen in the future, or obsessively rethinking a past mistake? Mindfulness, like healthy habit development, brings consciousness back into the picture by centering the practitioner in the present moment to cultivate well-being.

The goal of mindfulness is to extend or enhance what you know about yourself without judgment. In that sense, the mindfulness practices in the chapter work well with the recommendations in chapter 8. You can use your enhanced attention to determine what kind of self-care habits you might need.

Practicing mindfulness offers a multitude of benefits. It can help reduce stress, enhance the amount of information you can retain in your working memory, lessen the intensity of stress felt in interpersonal conflicts, and regulate mood. The physical sensation that accompanies practicing mindfulness has been described as feeling grounded, centered, or "in one's body." Biological benefits include better immunity and improved cardiac health. Emotional benefits such as preventing depression and reducing anxiety have also been found. Interpersonally, it may help increase feelings of connection.

In my own experience, I have seen my clients experience multiple benefits after engaging in mindful practices like the ones I will detail in this chapter.

Building Healthier Habits

Mindfulness can be incorporated into every experience. Throughout this chapter, the goal will be to reacquaint you with yourself, the actions you take, and the people you engage with. Although I will use the word deepen (as in "deepen your relationship") to describe this process, a client once described it as expanding from a two-dimensional perception of herself to a three-dimensional, fully realized view.

Mindfulness can help you reevaluate your relationship with time by making each moment count rather than maximizing the moments as they occur. The cliché of only having "this moment" sometimes obscures a deeper truth. While you carry your memories with you, you are not condemned to repeat any past mistake, just as, if you decide to, you can become the captain of your fate. But first you must not let your ability to have memories of the past or plans for the future take away the fact that each breath we take is a gift to appreciate.

Have Mindful Conversations

It's not uncommon to multitask while conversing with others—engaging in housework while talking with your kids or thinking about the errands you need to run while having a conversation with a coworker. Leaving the phone on the table while dining with friends so that you can quickly respond when a notification goes off is another example. Phones can be a significant obstacle to mindfulness.

You can build the habit of bringing more awareness to your interactions with the people in your life by limiting distractions from your moments of connection. To begin developing this habit, start with a commitment to not use your phone while having a face-to-face conversation.

1. The next time you are with a friend or family member, give them your full attention.
2. Place your phone out of reach and with the screen not visible.
3. When you have an urge to pick up the phone, tell yourself, "Don't do it."
4. Gently bring your focus back to the conversation.

Notice how much easier it is to respond and how easily the conversation flows because you haven't missed details due to distraction. You will likely gain a feeling of connection to people in your life as a result.

Helpful Tips:

→ If possible, when conversing, put your phone on mute.

→ To keep yourself from scrolling or using apps while you're talking on the phone with someone, place the phone facedown on the table and use its speaker phone function or earphones instead of holding it in your hands.

→ You can easily apply these strategies to your interactions with people you encounter in everyday situations, like the cashier while checking out at the grocery store. Focus on your interaction.

Mindful Bathing

Since bathing is a regular and necessary task, it is something that often gets rushed. Slowing down and making it a singular experience, in which you connect to your body and your senses, can be a physical reminder that you are giving yourself and your body care.

In developing this habit, you will practice mindful bathing by simply noticing what the water feels like on your skin. You might also pay attention to the sounds of the water or the scent of the soap you're using.

1. About two and a half hours before you go to bed, draw a bath or take a shower.
2. Commit to appreciating the feelings of bathing before you get into the water.
3. Revel in the sound and temperature of the water.
4. Appreciate the feeling of soap on your skin and other sensations you may be feeling.
5. When you have a random thought, let it float away and gently bring your attention back to bathing.
6. Relish the feeling of rinsing the soap away.
7. Embrace the feeling of air on your skin as you dry yourself off.

By practicing this habit, you will bring thoughtful attention to yourself, and by mindfully experiencing the moment that you're in, you will gain the ability to cast off distraction and, thus, gain a sense of relaxation and calm.

→ If this activity is uncomfortable, you might prefer to adjust it to mindful hand washing. To do so, extend the time washing your hands by a few seconds and bring your attention to the water, soap, sound, etc.

→ Use soap that has a pleasing aroma to add to the experience.

Wake Mindfully

I once heard Debbie Rosas, who is the founder of a dance and movement method called Nia, describe her morning ritual. Each morning, before she gets out of the bed or sits up, she stretches and moves her body to gently ease into the day. She encouraged the audience to adopt similar habits and, in essence, warm up before getting their morning started. We will draw from this great example of mindful waking by putting a slightly different spin on it.

The goal is to bring greater awareness to your body through a body scan. A body scan is the process of consciously drawing your attention to each area of your body. You focus on major areas of the body, starting at the crown of your head and slowly moving down to the soles of your feet, or vice versa. This can take as little as 10 seconds.

1. Upon waking, take three deep breaths.
2. Do a body scan and let each day guide you as to how long your scan takes.
3. If you feel any tightness, you can stretch or massage that area. Do another body scan, and notice any differences in your body.
4. Get out of bed and continue with your day.

This habit will strengthen your ability to give your body mindful attention throughout the day. You will likely notice that, without planning, you begin to stretch and massage areas that become tight during the day, leading to a more relaxed body.

→ An added benefit of the body scan is that it can help you notice what your body needs that day. Perhaps the rigorous exercise class you have planned would be better for another day and some gentle yoga is more what your body needs. What you glean from the body scan can help inform the self-care practices you focus on during a given day.

Monitor Negative Thoughts

Sometimes when you have negative or painful thoughts and judgments, you can begin to believe that, in some way, those thoughts define you. Instead, consider that you are the observer of your thoughts—you are not defined by them. Mindfulness helps you recognize and distinguish between the two. You are not, for example, an anxious person; you are a person experiencing anxiety or someone who has anxious thoughts.

Mindfulness makes space for you to observe those thoughts without attaching judgment or value to them; rather, you allow them to be like a leaf floating through your line of sight. In doing so, you might find that the power of those negative thoughts is reduced or at least comes into question.

1. When you next have a negative thought, remind yourself that you are an observer and not a judge.

2. Label it as a "thought." Repeat to yourself, "It's just a thought."

3. Bring your attention to your breath and calm your body.

4. Continue what you were doing when you noticed the thought.

5. Repeat as needed.

As this habit becomes ingrained, you will likely notice that you have gained some distance from or perspective on your thoughts. This may result in improved self-image, increased self-confidence, a greater sense of calm, or increased life satisfaction.

Helpful Tip:

→ Since you have many thoughts circulating in your head throughout the day, you may be alarmed by the number of negative thoughts you have. Stack this habit with ones from chapter 8 so that you can gently redirect your thoughts rather than become consumed by them.

Breaking Bad Habits

We live in a complex world, and our bodies are receiving and processing tons of stimuli of varying degrees of importance every day. It's remarkable that our brains and our senses can take in and process all of this while we attend to the living of our daily lives. But it's not surprising that, with everything bombarding us, it can be challenging sometimes to focus more singularly on the things that are important. When it becomes overly challenging, a common—though largely unconscious—coping habit is disconnection from the world. This is a bad habit because it limits the ability to see solutions and take advantage of new opportunities.

To break habits like this one, it's important to be mindfully connected to the solutions that exist in the present by reestablishing focus and balance. When you break habits that disconnect you from the world in the present, you will be better able to see beauty in moments of silence, connect with and engage in what you're doing, and bring greater awareness to new experiences.

Feeling Discomfort with Silence

Being in silence, even for short periods, can be uncomfortable. Western cultures have normalized filling gaps in conversation, lest the silence go on too long. Many people have accepted this norm, sometimes to the point of becoming uncomfortable with silence even when they are by themselves.

In therapy settings, it's important to allow for silence. Disturbing the norm allows space for the client to observe and process their thoughts so therapeutic material can emerge. Similarly, spending time with yourself in silence can bring a renewed awareness to your thoughts and increase your comfort of being with yourself undistracted. It can also give your brain a rest and make space for spontaneous ideas to arise.

1. Pick any five-minute stretch in your day to practice this habit, and set a recurring reminder to let you know it is time to begin. Turn off any external sounds (e.g., television, computer, phone ringer) around you.

2. Set your clock for five minutes and press start.

3. Sit in silence until the timer goes off.

4. Focus on your breath.

5. When the timer goes off, congratulate yourself by saying, "I did it."

6. Notice how you feel after allowing yourself to take this time.

Helpful Tips:

→ If there is no way to silence all of the sounds around you, just focus on what you have control over, like your breathing.

→ This is likely to be uncomfortable the first several times, but just bring your attention back to your breath.

→ Eventually, as your comfort increases, add time in 5-minute increments until you reach 20 minutes.

Rushing through Chores

It's easy to rush through everyday tasks so you can check them off your list and move on. This is especially true for household chores that you might not enjoy. But when you barrel through unpleasant things, you tune out and intensify the negative emotions attached to them, sapping your energy for future endeavors.

Instead of fighting the experience, I invite you to engage with it and yourself through mindfulness. In the book *The Miracle of Mindfulness* by Thích Nhất Hạnh, there is an entire passage extolling the virtues of dish washing. In it, the author describes the sense of aliveness that comes with fully immersing yourself in the experience of seemingly mundane tasks.

For this habit, I will use sweeping as the chore, but you can substitute any mundane, repetitive task that you want to focus on. Your job is to complete the task slowly and to pay attention to the experience rather than tuning out and disconnecting.

1. When the time comes for you to sweep, begin by noticing the sensation of holding the broom in your hand.

2. Listen to the sound the bristles make as they move across the floor.

3. Notice the particles on the floor. What colors do you see?

4. Feel your muscles as you move your arms back and forth.

5. Savor the emotion you have as you look at your clean floor.

Helpful Tips:
→ At any point that you find yourself rushing, say "Slow down," silently to yourself.

→ If you happen to enjoy all manner of household chores, substitute any regular activity you don't enjoy.

Getting Stuck in a Rut

Getting stuck in a rut is very similar to getting stuck in a bad habit loop, in that the bad habit loop involves actions that are very often unconscious and provide superficial or short-term gains that keep you disconnected from the things that matter. Having new and unique experiences is a way to get yourself out of a rut and make a conscious reconnection with the things that are important to you.

I invite you to try new micro-experiences to heighten your awareness through mindfulness. Think of some easily accessible experiences that you would like to try, like eating a new cuisine, visiting a nearby town, or even wearing a new color. Keep that list handy to customize the steps below to your liking. Here, I will share an example for taking a walk in a new neighborhood.

1. Identify one day of the week for an hour of exploration.

2. Upon arriving on the main street of the neighborhood, notice what is appealing and what is not. Do you like the architecture, the colors, the landscaping?

3. Check in with all your senses and savor the experience. Notice what you are curious about.

4. Take in and process what you feel about having this new experience.

5. Congratulate yourself for trying something new.

Helpful Tips:

→ As always, go somewhere where you feel safe and at a time of day that you will be safe.

→ To adapt this exercise, focus on noticing what is different.

Tracking Your Progress

Use this tracker as a tool to help you monitor your progress and gain insight into why a habit perhaps isn't quite sticking. We track our habits so we can learn, modify, and improve.

HABIT	M	T	W	TH	F	SAT	S

KEY TAKEAWAYS

- Mindfulness is the simple act of holding your experiences in your awareness without becoming too attached to them.

- Mindfulness is an approach to life, and as such, any activity in your life can become a mindful activity.

- You can strengthen the presence of mindfulness in your life in easy ways that can take seconds, minutes, or hours. The strategies in this chapter can be adjusted as you see fit.

- Practicing mindfulness is an important aspect of self-care that doesn't require you to change your life, but rather, to be more present in the one you have.

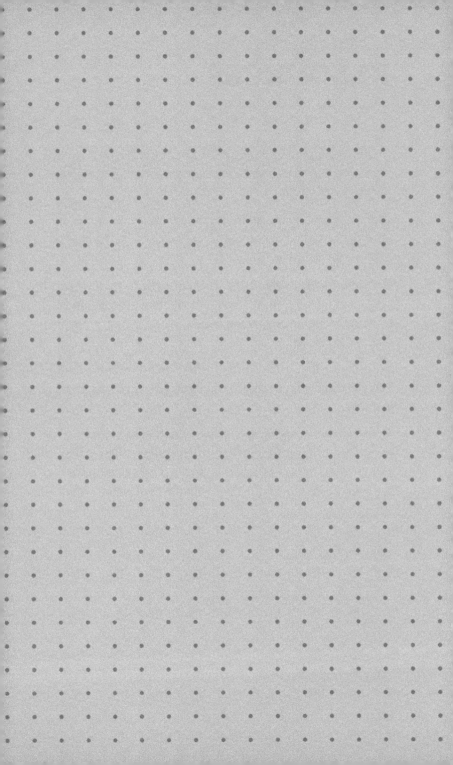

RESOURCES

@Womazeapp on Instagram: This account run by a family of mental health and self-care advocates is full of inspiration and validation.

@drcicelybrathwaite on Instagram: My account features information about how to improve your well-being at work and in your daily life.

GreaterGood.Berkeley.edu: Visit this website for all things related to well-being. You will find quizzes, articles, and podcasts that teach you the science of well-being in a fun and engaging way.

Mindful.org: Enjoy this website and sign up for the newsletter to gain access to mindfulness activities and insights.

PositivePsychology.com: This website has all kinds of resources to support your well-being based on positive psychology resources and research. Of particular note are their guides to progressive muscle relaxation.

Happify: This app is full of research-based positive psychology exercises and short courses designed to teach you skills to improve your mood.

Headspace: If you would like to try guided meditation, this app is a great place to begin. Users start with short meditations and move to longer ones as they gain more comfort with meditation.

Shine: This app contains meditations, sleep hygiene support, and guidance for developing self-care rituals led by women of color.

CicelyBrathwaite.com: To keep in touch, visit my website for my blog and learn about my self-care coaching and workshops.

All the Joy You Can Stand: 101 Sacred Power Principles for Making Joy Real in Your Life by Debrena Jackson Gandy: This classic text provides a useful foundation for developing a holistic approach to increasing joy.

REFERENCES

"11 Scientific Benefits of Being Outdoors." Mental Floss. November 2, 2015. www.mentalfloss.com/article/70548/11-scientific-benefits-being-outdoors.

"APA: U.S. Adults Report Highest Stress Level since Early Days of the COVID-19 Pandemic." American Psychological Association. Accessed March 1, 2021. www.apa.org/news/press/releases/2021/02/adults-stress-pandemic.

Beck, Melinda. "The Sleepless Elite." *The Wall Street Journal*. April 5, 2011. www.wsj.com/articles/SB10001424052748703712504576242701752957910.

Bratman, Gregory N., J. Paul Hamilton, Kevin S. Hahn, Gretchen C. Daily, and James J. Gross. "Nature Experience Reduces Rumination and Subgenual Prefrontal Cortex Activation." *Proceedings of the National Academy of Sciences* 112, no. 28 (July 2015): 8567–72. doi.org/10.1073/pnas.1510459112.

Brown, Brené. *Braving the Wilderness: The Quest for True Belonging and the Courage to Stand Alone*. New York: Random House, 2019.

Capaldi, Colin, Raelyne Dopko, and John Zelenski. "The Relationship between Nature Connectedness and Happiness: A Meta-Analysis." *Frontiers in*

Psychology 5 (September 2014). doi.org/10.3389
/fpsyg.2014.00976.

Crego, Adam C., Fabián Štoček, Alec G. Marchuk,
James E. Carmichael, Matthijs A. van der Meer, and
Kyle S. Smith. "Complementary Control over
Habits and Behavioral Vigor by Phasic Activity in the
Dorsolateral Striatum." *The Journal of Neuroscience*
40, no. 10 (March 2020): 2139–53. doi.org/10.1523/
jneurosci.1313-19.2019.

Dalton-Smith, Saundra. *Sacred Rest: Recover Your Life,
Renew Your Energy, Restore Your Sanity.* New York: Faith
Words, 2019.

Davis, Daphne M. "What Are the Benefits of Mindfulness."
Monitor on Psychology. American Psychological Association. Accessed February 21, 2021. www.apa.org
/monitor/2012/07-08/ce-corner.

Duhigg, Charles. *The Power of Habit: Why We Do What We Do
in Life and Business.* Toronto: Anchor Canada, 2014.

Foerde, Karin. "What Are Habits and Do They Depend on
the Striatum? A View from the Study of Neuropsy-
chological Populations." *Current Opinion in Behavioral
Sciences* 20 (April 2018): 17–24. doi.org/10.1016/j
.cobeha.2017.08.011.

Geronimus, Arline T., Margaret Hicken, Danya Keene,
and John Bound. "'Weathering' and Age Patterns of
Allostatic Load Scores Among Blacks and Whites in
the United States." *American Journal of Public Health* 96,
no. 5 (May 2006): 826–33. doi.org/10.2105/ajph.2004
.060749.

Gonzalo, Angelo, "Dorothea Orem: Self-Care Deficit Theory Study Guide." Nurseslabs. August 24, 2019. nurseslabs.com/dorothea-orems-self-care-theory/.

Graybiel, Ann M., and Scott T. Grafton. "The Striatum: Where Skills and Habits Meet." *Cold Spring Harbor Perspectives in Biology* 7, no. 8 (August 2015). doi.org /10.1101/cshperspect.a021691.

Hạnh, Thích Nhất. *The Miracle of Mindfulness: An Introduction to the Practice of Meditation*. Translated by Mobi Ho. Boston: Beacon Press, 2016.

Hermanto, Nicola, and David Charles Zuroff. "The Social Mentality Theory of Self-Compassion and Self-Reassurance: The Interactive Effect of Care-Seeking and Caregiving." *Journal of Social Psychology* 156, no. 5 (September/October 2016): 523–35. doi.org/10.1080/00224545.2015.1135779.

"How to Get a Great Nap." Mayo Clinic. Mayo Foundation for Medical Education and Research. November 13, 2020. www.mayoclinic.org/healthy-lifestyle/adult -health/in-depth/napping/art-20048319.

"Identify Your Habit Loops: The Basic Structure Behind Every Single Habit." The Emotion Machine. November 30, 2020. www.theemotionmachine.com/habit-loops/.

Kaimal, Girija, Hasan Ayaz, Joanna Herres, Rebekka Dieterich-Hartwell, Bindal Makwana, Donna H. Kaiser, and Jennifer A. Nasser. "Functional Near-Infrared Spectroscopy Assessment of Reward Perception

Based on Visual Self-Expression: Coloring, Doo-dling, and Free Drawing." *The Arts in Psychotherapy* 55 (September 2017): 85–92. doi.org/10.1016/j .aip.2017.05.004.

Keller, Jan, Dominika Kwasnicka, Patrick Klaiber, Lena Sichert, Phillippa Lally, and Lena Fleig. "Habit For-mation Following Routine-Based versus Time-Based Cue Planning: A Randomized Controlled Trial." *British Journal of Health Psychology* (January 2021). doi.org/10.1111/bjhp.12504.

Kim, S. H., Y. H. Kim, and H. J. Kim. "Laughter and Stress Relief in Cancer Patients: A Pilot Study." *Evidence-Based Complementary and Alternative Medicine* (May 2015): 1–6. doi.org/10.1155/2015/864739.

Kohll, Alan. "New Study Shows Correlation between Employee Engagement and the Long-Lost Lunch Break." *Forbes*. May 30, 2018. www.forbes.com /sites/alankohll/2018/05/29/new-study-shows -correlation-between-employee-engagement -and-the-long-lost-lunch-break.

Smith, Kyle S. "Habit Formation." *Dialogues in Clinical Neuroscience* 18, no. 1 (2016): 33–43. https://doi. org/10.31887/dcns.2016.18.1/ksmith.

Lawton, Emma, Eric Brymer, Peter Clough, and Andrew Denovan. "The Relationship between the Physical Activity Environment, Nature Relatedness, Anxiety, and the Psychological Well-Being Benefits of Regular

Exercisers." *Frontiers in Psychology* 8 (June 2017). doi.org/10.3389/fpsyg.2017.01058.

"MIT Researcher Sheds Light on Why Habits Are Hard to Make and Break." MIT News | Massachusetts Institute of Technology. Accessed March 2, 2021. news.mit .edu/1999/habits.

Nagoski, Emily, and Amelia Nagoski. *Burnout: The Secret to Unlocking the Stress Cycle*. New York: Ballantine Books, 2020.

"Napping: Health Benefits & Tips for Your Best Nap." Sleep Foundation. October 9, 2020. www.sleepfoundation .org/sleep-hygiene/napping.

Neff, Kristin. "Self-Compassion: An Alternative Conceptualization of a Healthy Attitude Toward Oneself." *Self and Identity* 2, no. 2 (April 2003): 85–101. doi.org /10.1080/15298860309032.

Nureeva, Liliya, Karen Brunsø, and Liisa Lähteenmäki. "Exploring Self-Regulatory Strategies for Eating Behaviour in Danish Adolescents." *Young Consumers* 17, no. 2 (June 2016): 155–67. doi.org/10.1108/yc-10 -2015-00565.

Olson, Deborah. *Success The Psychology of Achievement*. London: Dorling Kindersley Limited, 2017.

Quinn, Jeffrey M., Anthony Pascoe, Wendy Wood, and David T. Neal. "Can't Control Yourself? Monitor Those Bad Habits." *Personality and Social Psychology Bulletin* 36, no. 4 (April 2010): 499–511. doi.org/10.1177 /0146167209360665.

Ramírez-Vizcaya, Susana, and Tom Froese. "The Enactive Approach to Habits: New Concepts for the Cognitive Science of Bad Habits and Addiction." Frontiers. January 30, 2019. www.frontiersin.org/articles /10.3389/fpsyg.2019.00301/full.

Rees, Amelia, Mark W. Wiggins, William S. Helton, Thomas Loveday, and David O'Hare. "The Impact of Breaks on Sustained Attention in a Simulated, Semi-Automated Train Control Task." *Applied Cognitive Psychology* 31, no. 3 (May 2017): 351–59. doi.org/10.1002/acp.3334.

Riopel, Leslie. "15 Most Interesting Self-Compassion Research Findings (Incl. Theory)." Positive Psychology. Accessed February 27, 2021. positivepsychology .com/self-compassion-research/.

Rubin, Gretchen. "Want to Change an Important Habit? Tips for Upholders, Questioners, Obligers & Rebels." *Gretchen Ruben* (blog). Accessed March 2, 2021. gretchenrubin.com/2017/07/want-to-change -an-important-habit/.

Seligman, Martin E. P. *Flourish: The New Positive Psychology and the Search for Well-Being*. New York: Free Press, 2011.

"Spend Time in Nature to Reduce Stress and Anxiety." American Heart Association. Accessed March 21, 2021. www.heart.org/en/healthy-living/healthy -lifestyle/stress-management/spend-time-in-nature -to-reduce-stress-and-anxiety.

The Greater Good Science Center at the University of California, Berkeley. "Social Connection Defined."

Greater Good Magazine. Accessed April 15, 2021.
greatergood.berkeley.edu/topic/social_connection
/definition#what-is-social-connection.

Thorpe, Matthew. "12 Benefits of Meditation." Healthline.
October 27, 2020. www.healthline.com/nutrition
/12-benefits-of-meditation.

White, Mathew P., Ian Alcock, James Grellier, Benedict
W. Wheeler, Terry Hartig, Sara L. Warber, Angie Bone,
Michael H. Depledge, and Lora E. Fleming. "Spending
at Least 120 Minutes a Week in Nature Is Associated
with Good Health and Wellbeing." *Scientific Reports* 9,
no. 1 (June 2019). doi.org/10.1038/s41598-019
-44097-3.

Wu, Chunxiao, Qu Yi, Xiaoyan Zheng, Shaoyang Cui,
Bin Chen, Liming Lu, and Chunzhi Tang. "Effects of
Mind-Body Exercises on Cognitive Function in Older
Adults: A Meta-Analysis." *Journal of the American
Geriatrics Society* 67, no. 4 (April 2018): 749–58.
doi.org/10.1111/jgs.15714.

INDEX

T

U

V

W

Z

Acknowledgments

Dr. Charles N. Jamison Jr., you demonstrate daily what self-care habits look like. Barbara McFadden and Steve Horsham-Brathwaite, thanks for being my parents and for instilling in me a thirst for knowledge. I love you.

To my siblings, Lisa Tyson-Brathwaite and Desmond Horsham-Brathwaite, your resilience and care amaze me.

To my aunties, uncles, and cousins, all my love. Taylor, Kennedy, and Makenzie, keep shining! Tiffany, thank you for blessing me with loving and brilliant goddaughters.

Dr. Darien McFadden, all I ever wanted was to be like you. Thank you for bringing psychology into my life. Dr. Portia Hunt and Dr. Sharon Kirkland-Gordon, how can I thank you enough for all that you taught me?

June, Marquita, Alex, Janine, and Nini, I am grateful for your friendship.

About the Author

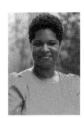 **Cicely Horsham-Brathwaite, PhD,** is a licensed counseling psychologist, executive coach, and organizational consultant with more than two decades of experience. She is a passionate advocate for self-care in her personal life and professional practice. She has been featured on the BBC World Service and in *HuffPost*, *SELF*, *Entrepreneur*, and *CNBC Make It*.

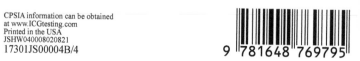

9 781648 769795